Applied equine nutrition

Applied equine nutrition

Equine NUtrition COnference (ENUCO) 2005

edited by:

A. Lindner

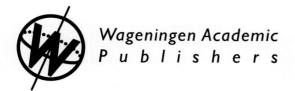

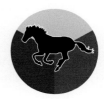

Subject headings:
Health
Disease
Horse

Photos cover: Derek Cuddeford and Arno Lindner

ISBN 907699885X
ISBN 300016376X

First published, 2005

Wageningen Academic Publishers The Netherlands, 2005

Table of contents

Editorial

It is a great pleasure to have run the first Equine NUtrition COnference (ENUCO) in Hannover, Germany, on October 1 and 2, 2005. I strongly believe that there is a need for disseminating scientifically validated knowledge for practitioners, and that there can not be enough seminars, conferences and courses to achieve this. This book will aid in propagating the information too. In addition, scientists as a group need to get, as often as possible, in contact with practitioners, to focus their research and improve networking. ENUCO provides such an opportunity too.

Both objectives could not have been realized without the financial and ideological partnership offered by Alltech, Life Data Labs, Lohmann Animal Health/Lonza and Plantavet. Thank you!

Wish you a benefit from the contents of this book!

Arno Lindner

Digestibility and retention of inorganic and organic forms of copper and zinc in yearling and mature geldings*

Lance A. Baker
Equine Industry Program, West Texas A&M University, Canyon, TX, USA

Introduction

A mineral proteinate is a chelated mineral complex that is formed by reacting a mineral salt with a specifically prepared mixture of amino acids and small peptides. The chelate that results from the binding of the mineral and amino acid carries no electrical charge, and remains stable in the presence of pH changes in the gastrointestinal tract. Because of this electrical neutrality, the mineral in organic complex form is theorized to be more bioavailable to the animal, and utilize a different absorptive mechanism than a mineral in its "natural" or inorganic state. Numerous studies in rats, poultry, pigs, and ruminants have shown an increased bioavailability of the mineral proteinate as compared to the inorganic form. Recently, several studies have reported varying results with regard to the digestibility and retention of inorganic and organic forms of Cu and Zn.

Objectives

The objective of these trials was to determine the effects of supplemental inorganic and organic forms of Cu and Zn on digestibility and daily balance (or retention) in yearling geldings in training (Phase I) and mature, sedentary geldings (Phase II).

---
*This paper was selected to be presented at ENUCO-Practice 2005 from the presentations at the Conference of the Equine Science Society (ESS) held in Tucson, Arizona, USA, in May/June 2005.

Materials and methods

Phase I

Twelve yearling stock-type geldings were stratified by weight and randomly assigned to one of three diets: control, inorganic or organic Cu and Zn supplemented. The trial consisted of four 30-d experimental periods with 72-h collection periods at the end of each period. Total urine and fecal collections were taken during the 72-h collection periods. Blood samples, and radiographs were taken the first morning of each collection period. Beginning on d 50, all horses were placed on an identical exercise regime consisting of 15 min non-circular longeing at the trot. Horses were fed individually at 12-h intervals, provided fresh water *ad libitum*, and allowed 2 to 4 h to consume their respective ration before being turned out in a dry lot each day. Radiographs were scanned at the nutrient foramen of the third metacarpal (front cannon bone) with a Bio-Rad Model 620 Densitometer to determine bone density. A logarithmic regression was formed using the thickness of steps on an aluminum penetrometer to determine the radiographic bone aluminum equivalence (RBAE) from the maximal optical density readings of both cortices for each view of the metacarpal.

Diets were formulated to meet or exceed NRC requirements and to reflect mineral supplementation common to the equine industry for yearlings in training at moderate growth. Concentrates were fed with matua-alfalfa hay in a 65:35 grain to hay ratio. The concentrate diets were formulated using a base concentrate of corn, soybean meal, cottonseed hulls, and dehydrated alfalfa meal. The control diet (C) contained no supplemental Cu or Zn. The inorganic Cu and Zn supplemented concentrate (IM) was formulated to contain approximately 50 ppm Cu and 200 ppm Zn by adding $CuSO_4$ and ZnO. The organic Cu and Zn supplemented concentrate (OM) was formulated by replacing 45% of the supplemented inorganic minerals with Alltech's Bioplex© Cu and Zn (Alltech Biotechnology, Inc., Lexington, KY). Concentrate formulation and concentrate and hay analyses are shown in Tables 1, 2, and 3, respectively. Statistical analyses were conducted using repeated measures within the General Linear Models procedure, with treatment and time as main effects; time as the repeated variable; and all interactions (SAS, 2000). Due to the unavoidable and unrelated death of two geldings, one each from IM and OM creating unequal data groups, least square means were calculated to compare means (C, n = 4; IM,

Table 1. Concentrate formulation, phase I.

Ingredient, unit	Control	Inorganic	Organic
Ground shelled corn, %	61.0	61.0	61.0
44% CP soybean meal, %	15.0	15.0	15.0
Cottonseed hulls, %	10.0	10.0	10.0
Dehydrated alfalfa, %	6.5	6.5	6.5
Soybean oil, %	3.0	3.0	3.0
Liquid molasses, %	2.0	2.0	2.0
Trace mineralized Salt, %	1.0	1.0	1.0
Limestone, %	1.0	1.0	1.0
Dicalcium phosphate, %	0.5	0.5	0.5
Copper sulfate, g/ton	–	144.3	79.4
Zinc oxide, g/ton	–	202.1	111.1
Bioplex copper[a], g/ton	–	–	164.0
Bioplex zinc[a], g/ton	–	–	437.0

[a]Alltech Biotechnology, Inc., Lexington, KY

Table 2. Concentrate analysis (phase I, dry matter basis).

Ingredient, units	Control	Inorganic	Organic
Moisture, %	7.0	7.1	7.1
CP, %	14.2	13.6	13.8
ADF, %	14.0	13.9	13.0
Ash, %	1.3	3.1	3.3
Ether extract, %	6.5	6.9	5.6
Ca, %	0.7	0.7	0.7
P, %	0.4	0.4	0.3
Cu, ppm	23.4	51.2	61.0
Zn, ppm	66.6	189.9	216.6

n = 3; OM, n = 3). Non-orthogonal contrasts were used to determine differences between time means (d 30 vs d 60, 90, and 120). Orthogonal contrasts were used to determine differences between treatment means (C vs the mean of IM and OM, and IM vs OM).

Table 3. Matua-alfalfa analysis (phase I, dry matter basis).

Ingredient, units	Quantity
Moisture, %	14.0
CP, %	13.5
ADF, %	31.2
Ash, %	13.1
Ether extract, %	2.6
Ca, %	0.8
P, %	0.2
Cu, ppm	35.1
Zn, ppm	29.5

Phase II

Nine mature horses 12 to 18 yr of age, were randomly divided into three groups and placed on either a control (C), organically chelated (OM) or inorganic (IM) Cu and Zn-added diet within three simultaneous 3x3 Latin Square design experiments. The trial consisted of three 28-d experimental periods consisting of a 25-d feed adjustment period followed by a 72-h collection period. Total urine and feces were collected during the 72-h collection period and analyzed for Cu and Zn concentrations using standard flame atomic absorption spectrophotometric methodology. Venous blood samples were drawn the first morning of each collection period. Horses were fed individually at 12-h intervals, provided fresh water *ad libitum*, and allowed 2 to 4 h to consume their ration before being turned out. Diets were formulated to meet or exceed NRC (1989) requirements for mature horses performing light work. Concentrates were fed with prairie grass hay in a 60:40 grain to hay ratio. The control diet (C) contained no supplemented Cu or Zn. The IM diet was supplemented with approximately 40 ppm Cu and 160 ppm Zn by adding $CuSO_4$ and ZnO. The OM diet was formulated by replacing 45% of the supplemented inorganic minerals with Alltech's Bioplex® Cu and Zn (Alltech Biotechnology, Inc., Lexington, KY). Concentrate and hay analyses are

Table 4. Concentrate analysis (phase II, dry matter basis).

Nutrient, units	C	IM	OM
Moisture, %	8.69	7.90	8.50
CP, %	10.41	10.73	10.16
ADF, %	21.11	21.07	21.66
Ash, %	5.37	5.84	5.34
Ether extract, %	3.77	3.45	3.45
Cu, ppm	6.68	66.60	52.97
Zn, ppm	72.27	373.67	304.58

Table 5. Hay analysis (phase II, dry matter basis).

Nutrient, units	Quantity
Moisture, %	5.71
CP, %	6.50
ADF, %	43.96
Ash, %	5.49
Ether extract, %	1.33
Cu, ppm	4.77
Zn, ppm	33.58

shown in Tables 4 and 5, respectively. Statistical analyses were conducted using the General Linear Models analysis of variance procedure to determine main effects of treatment, period, and horse. Duncan's Multiple Range Test was used to determine differences between treatment means with significant differences declared at $P < 0.05$ (SAS, 2000).

Results and discussion

Phase I

Horses consuming OM had a greater mean apparent daily Cu balance ($P < 0.001$; Figure 1), balance as a percent of intake ($P < 0.001$; Figure

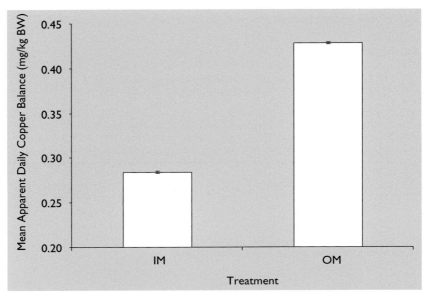

Figure 1. The effect of treatment (IM vs OM) on mean apparent daily Cu balance in yearling geldings over 120 d (P < 0.001).

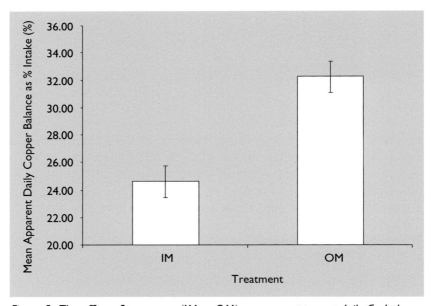

Figure 2. The effect of treatment (IM vs OM) on mean apparent daily Cu balance as a percent of intake in yearling geldings over 120 d (P < 0.001).

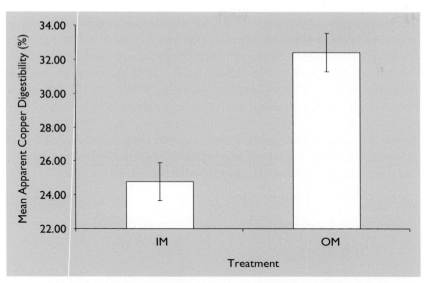

Figure 3. The effect of treatment (IM vs OM) on mean apparent Cu digestibility in yearling geldings over 120 d (P < 0.001).

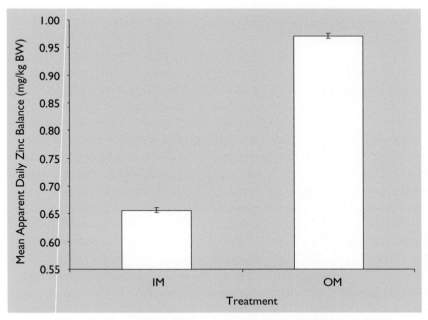

Figure 4. The effect of treatment (IM vs OM) on mean apparent daily Zn balance in yearling geldings over 120 d (P < 0.001).

2), and apparent digestibility (P < 0.001; Figure 3) as compared to horses consuming IM. Horses consuming OM had a greater mean apparent daily Zn balance (P < 0.001; Figure 4) as compared to horses consuming IM. There was no difference (P < 0.792) between Cu sources on mean serum Cu concentration (Table 6). There was no difference between Zn sources on mean serum Zn concentration (P < 0.634; Table

Table 6. Mean daily Cu intake, fecal and urinary excretion; apparent daily balance, balance as a percent of intake, and balance as a percent of absorption; apparent digestibility; and serum concentration in yearling geldings for all treatments over 120 d.

Item, Unit		Time (Days)			
		30	60	90	120
Cu intake, mg/kg BW	Control	0.69	0.70	0.69	0.69
	Inorganic	1.15	1.16	1.15	1.15
	Organic	1.35	1.32	1.32	1.32
Fecal Cu, mg/kg BW	Control	0.36	0.33	0.42	0.42
	Inorganic	0.72	0.88	1.00	0.88
	Organic	0.79	0.89	1.04	0.87
Urine Cu, ug/kg BW	Control	1.58	1.71	1.94	2.02
	Inorganic	1.72	2.73	2.27	1.92
	Organic	1.67	2.17	2.20	2.25
Cu balance, mg/kg BW	Control	0.34	0.36	0.27	0.27
	Inorganic	0.43	0.27	0.16	0.27
	Organic	0.56	0.43	0.28	0.45
Cu balance as % intake, %	Control	48.50	52.00	38.41	38.66
	Inorganic	37.67	23.54	13.42	23.79
	Organic	41.52	32.43	20.89	34.06
Cu balance as % absorbed, %	Control	99.52	99.51	99.24	99.24
	Inorganic	99.59	99.02	98.22	99.29
	Organic	99.70	99.49	99.20	99.50
Cu digestibility, %	Control	48.73	52.24	38.69	38.96
	Inorganic	37.83	23.78	13.62	23.96
	Organic	41.64	32.60	21.06	34.23
Serum Cu, ppm	Control	1.31	1.26	1.08	1.10
	Inorganic	1.12	1.34	1.10	1.09
	Organic	1.18	1.41	1.04	1.10

Table 7. Mean daily Zn intake, fecal and urinary excretion; apparent daily balance, balance as a percent of intake, and balance as a percent of absorption; apparent digestibility; and serum concentration in yearling geldings for all treatments over 120 d.

Item, Unit		Time (Days)			
		30	60	90	120
Zn intake, mg/kg BW	Control	1.36	1.37	1.35	1.35
	Inorganic	3.42	3.40	3.39	3.38
	Organic	3.87	3.83	3.38	3.85
Fecal Zn, mg/kg BW	Control	1.10	1.10	1.13	1.16
	Inorganic	2.74	2.73	2.80	2.67
	Organic	2.87	2.95	3.06	2.59
Urine Zn, ug/kg BW	Control	9.06	7.59	5.37	6.23
	Inorganic	5.84	8.13	6.10	4.62
	Organic	7.60	8.64	6.36	5.31
Zn balance, mg/kg BW	Control	0.25	0.26	0.21	0.18
	Inorganic	0.67	0.66	0.58	0.71
	Organic	0.99	0.87	0.78	1.25
Zn balance as % intake, %	Control	18.26	19.16	15.73	13.06
	Inorganic	19.62	19.44	17.18	20.89
	Organic	25.66	22.76	20.23	32.39
Zn balance as % absorbed, %	Control	95.84	96.38	97.24	96.08
	Inorganic	98.98	98.41	98.73	99.33
	Organic	99.24	99.02	99.19	99.58
Zn Digestibility, %	Control	18.93	19.72	16.13	13.53
	Inorganic	19.85	19.68	17.36	21.03
	Organic	25.85	22.98	20.40	32.53
Serum Zn, ppm	Control	0.96	0.39	0.82	0.63
	Inorganic	0.94	0.47	0.84	0.64
	Organic	0.87	0.45	0.86	0.67

7). No differences due to treatment were detected in lateral, medial, palmar, or dorsal RBAE's at any time during the trial.

While the IM and OM concentrate diets were formulated to contain equivalent amounts of Cu and Zn, upon analysis, the OM concentrate contained 61 ppm Cu and 216 ppm Zn, while the IM concentrate contained 61 ppm Cu and 190 ppm Zn. Due to the resulting differences in Cu and Zn intake between OM and IM horses, it is important to weigh the daily balance (retention) data with the balance as a percent of intake data to compare the supplemental forms of the minerals. It is also interesting to note that the C concentrate contained 23 ppm Cu and 66 ppm Zn using standard ingredients, which are both well above NRC requirements for these minerals (10 ppm Cu, 40 ppm Zn). Apparent daily balance (or retention) data can sometimes be difficult to interpret in feeding trials. Oftentimes, as mineral intake increases above daily requirements, daily balance, or retention, also increases. A cursory glance at the balance data from this trial might lead one to conclude that this is the cause of the significantly higher daily Cu and Zn balance in those horses consuming the OM diet as compared to the IM diet (Figures 1 and 4), as intake of both minerals was higher for these horses. However, this is not the case with Cu, as daily Cu balance (or

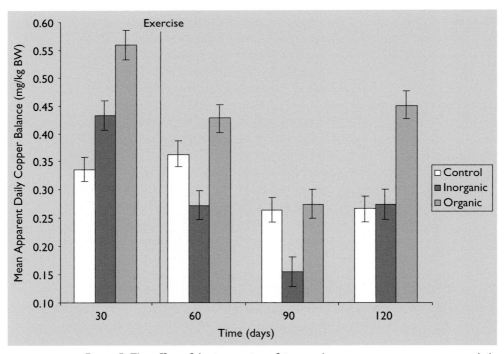

Figure 5. The effect of the interaction of time and treatment on mean apparent daily Cu balance in yearling geldings for all treatments over 120 d (P < 0.001).

retention) as a percent of intake (Figure 4) was also significantly higher for those consuming OM as compared to those consuming IM. As can be seen in Figure 5, apparent daily Cu balance (or retention) for those horses consuming both IM and OM appear to follow a very similar trend. Daily balances in both groups appear to decrease at day 60 and again at day 90, before increasing at day 120. This decrease and subsequent increase could be explained by the beginning of the exercise regimen on day 50 causing an increased need for Cu by various enzymes and/or the increased bone remodeling that is taking place. Another possible explanation for this trend is an immune response to disease and a subsequent depletion of body stores of Cu. Although all horses were vaccinated for *streptococcus equi* (strangles) upon arrival at the WTAMU Horse Center, all horses became symptomatic of strangles before the beginning of the trial, and continued to suffer mild symptoms through approximately day 100.

The digestibility data in Figure 6 provide further evidence for the effectiveness of the organically chelated Cu used in this study. As a general rule, mineral digestibility, as a percentage, tends to decrease as intake increases above the daily requirement. This theory holds true

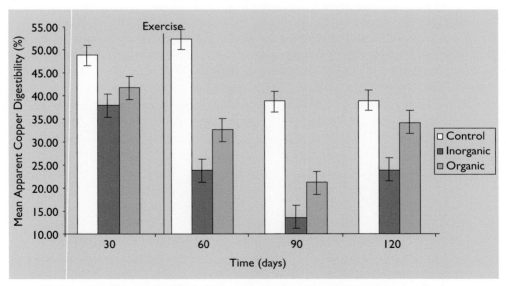

Figure 6. The effect of the interaction of time and treatment on mean apparent Cu digestibility in yearling geldings for all treatments over 120 d (P < 0.007).

with regard to horses consuming C as compared to both IM and OM (Figure 6). However, even though horses consuming OM were consuming more Cu as compared to horses consuming IM (1.32 vs. 1.15 mg/kg BW, respectively; Table 6), their Cu digestibility was higher at every time point measured (Figure 6), and was significantly higher overall (Figure 3).

No differences due to treatment were detected for Zn balance as a percent of intake or apparent Zn digestibility (Table 7). However, horses consuming OM had significantly higher apparent daily Zn balance (retention) as compared to horses consuming IM (Figure 4). This increased daily balance could be explained by a slightly higher Zn intake by horses consuming OM as compared to IM. However, as observed in the Cu data, this increase could be due to horses more efficiently retaining the organically chelated Zn used in this study.

Phase II

Apparent mean daily Cu digestibility was higher (P < 0.002) for horses consuming IM as compared to horses consuming OM and C (Figure 7). Wagner *et al.* (2003) reported no significant difference in Cu absorption in mature horses supplemented with oxide, sulfate, or organically

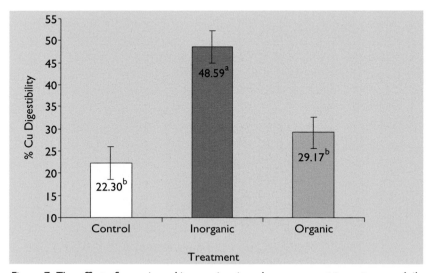

Figure 7. The effect of organic and inorganic mineral sources on apparent mean daily Cu digestibility in mature horses (P < 0.001).

chelated forms of Cu, possibly due to the age of the horses or a short feed adjustment period of 10 d.

Apparent mean daily Cu balance was greater (P < 0.001) for horses consuming IM as compared to horses consuming OM and C (Figure 8). Additionally, apparent mean daily Cu balance was higher (P < 0.001) for horses consuming OM as compared to horses consuming C. This agrees with Apgar and Kornegay (1996) who reported increased apparent absorption in pigs fed elevated Cu levels regardless of source, as compared to pigs fed control diets. Wagner *et al.* (2003) reported no significant difference in Cu retention in mature horses supplemented with oxide, sulfate, or organically chelated forms of Cu.

There was no main effect of treatment (P < 0.198) on mean apparent daily Zn digestibility (Figure 9). These results agree with Wagner *et al.* (2003) who reported no significant difference in apparent Zn absorption in mature horses supplemented with oxide, sulfate, or organically-chelated forms of Zn. The NRC (1989) states that apparent Zn absorption ranges from 5 to 10% in horses, while apparent Zn digestibility in the current study ranged from 28 to 35%. As animals age, a decrease in the digestibility of many nutrients occurs, however,

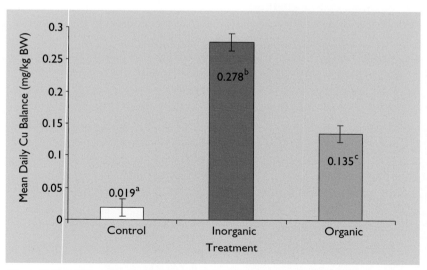

Figure 8. *The effect of organic and inorganic mineral sources on apparent mean daily Cu balance in mature horses (P < 0.001).*

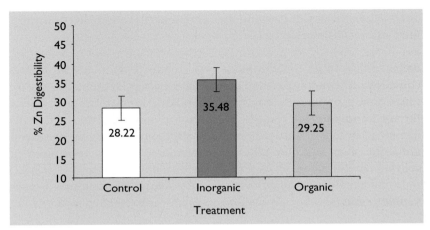

Figure 9. The effect of organic and inorganic mineral sources on apparent mean daily Zn digestibility in mature horses (P < 0.198).

there is conflicting evidence concerning the effect of age on Zn digestibility, as observed in a study on cattle where there was no effect on Zn digestibility between lactating cows and 2 to 6 mo old calves (Underwood, 1977). In several studies (Underwood, 1977, Miller *et al.*, 2003, Wagner *et al.*, 2003), there was no effect of Zn intake or source on apparent Zn digestibility.

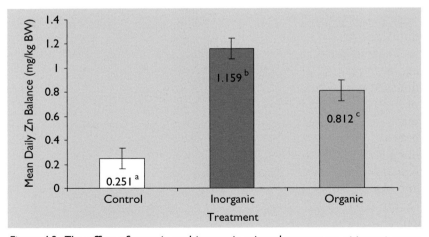

Figure 10. The effect of organic and inorganic mineral sources on apparent mean daily Zn balance in mature horses (P < 0.001).

Mean daily Zn balance was lower (P < 0.012) in horses consuming C as compared to horses consuming IM and OM (Figure 10). Additionally, daily Zn balance was greater (P < 0.012) for horses consuming IM as compared to horses consuming OM. This differs from Wagner *et al.* (2003) who reported no significant difference in Zn retention in mature horses supplemented with oxide, sulfate, or organically chelated forms of Zn. The differences in daily Zn balance may be explained by greater intakes of Zn in mature horses consuming the IM diet, and greater intakes of Zn in yearlings consuming the OM diet.

Conclusions

Results from Phase I indicate that yearling geldings supplemented with the organically chelated form of Cu and Zn (Alltech's Bioplex© Cu and Zn) had significantly higher Cu digestibilities, daily balance, and balance as a percent of intake, and significantly higher apparent daily Zn balance as compared to those supplemented with the inorganic form of these minerals.

Results from Phase II indicate that mature horses may utilize organic and inorganic sources of Cu and Zn differently than yearling horses. An increase in mean apparent daily Cu digestibility, and Cu and Zn balance was observed in horses consuming IM as compared to horses consuming OM and C. The reason that mature horses consuming organic minerals in both this trial and the trial by Wagner *et al.* (2003) did not respond as yearling horses in Phase I is unclear. However, there are many factors that may have contributed to these results, including age of the horses used and amounts of Cu and Zn in the IM and OM diets. Mature horses may also have a decreased ability to absorb proteinated minerals due to less efficient digestion of proteins, which may occur as the animal ages. Furthermore, the precise relationship between mineral intake and digestibility is unclear. There may be a non-linear digestibility response to intake for horses consuming Cu and Zn, which could account for the differences in digestibilities seen in these and other studies. Since feed manufacturers continue to supplement Cu and Zn in mature horse diets, the effect of supplemental Cu and Zn needs to be studied further.

References

Alltech, Inc. 2001. Introduction to the Bioplexes. Alltech, Inc. Biotechnology Center. Nicholasville, KY.

Apgar, G.A., and E.T. Kornegay. 1996. Mineral balance of finishing pigs fed copper sulfate or a copper-lysine complex at growth-stimulating levels. J. Anim. Sci. 74:1594-1600.

Baker L.A., T. Kearney-Moss, J.L. Pipkin, R.C. Bachman, J.T. Haliburton and G.O. Veneklasen. 2003. The Effect of Supplemental Inorganic and Organic Sources of Copper and Zinc on Bone Metabolism in Exercised Yearling Geldings. Proc. 18th Equine Nutr. And Physiol. Symp. East Lansing, MI. Pp 100-105.

Miller E.D., L.A. Baker, J.L. Pipkin, R.C. Bachman, J.T. Haliburton and G.O. Veneklasen. 2003. The Effect of Supplemental Inorganic and Organic Forms of Copper and Zinc on Digestibility in Yearling Geldings in Training. Proc. 18th Equine Nutr. And Physiol. Symp. East Lansing, MI. Pp 107-112.

NRC. 1989. Nutrient Requirement of Horses (5th Ed.). Nat'l Acad. Press, Washington, DC.

SAS. 2000. SAS User's Guide (Version 8.1). SAS Inst. Inc., Cary, NC

Underwood, E.J. 1977. Trace Elements in Human and Animal Nutrition. 4th ed. Academic Press, New York, NY.

Wagner, E.L., G.D. Potter, E.M. Michael, P.G. Gibbs and D.M. Hood. 2003. Absorption and Retention of Various Forms of Trace Minerals in Horses. Proc. 18th Equine Nutr. And Physiol. Symp. East Lansing, MI. Pp 26-30.

The impact of nutrition on dental health and management of equine teeth for optimal nutrition

Ian Dacre
IVABS, Massey University, Private Bag 11222, Palmerston North, New Zealand

Abstract

Equine dentition is a reflection of the diet to which it has evolved over the past 50-70 million years. Modern management and feeding practices have resulted in reduced wear to the occlusal table from decreased mastication, together with a reduction in lateral excursion of cheek teeth when horses are fed a high percentage of concentrate in their diet. This is the principle reason for the increased formation of sharp dental overgrowths in stabled horses. Limited studies looking at whether current dental procedures affect feed digestibility have shown excessive crown reduction to have a deleterious effect, whilst in a separate study dental pathology has been associated with low body condition score. Although not yet specifically linked in the horse, evidence exists that nutritional odontodystrophies may occur as already established for other species. The relationship between common dental pathology such as periodontal disease or caries and diet continues to be explored, however the link between oral health status and diet selection - an area already well established for humans - has yet to be investigated for equids.

Introduction

Dentition is a reflection of the diet to which it has evolved. Some 50-70 million years ago, the first member of the *Equidae* family (*Hyracotherium*) evolved with brachydont (short-crowned) dentition that was to further adapt following climate changes and corresponding changes to its herbivorous diet (Bennett, 1992). This change to a coarser, more abrasive and fibrous diet necessitated the development of more complex teeth. Incisors became specialised for efficient cropping of grass during prolonged periods of grazing of up to 16.5 hours per day (Budiansky, 1997; Capper, 1992). Occlusal crown wear during such long grazing periods is usually reported to be 2-3mm per year in the modern horse, however crown loss may actually be as high as 7-8mm per annum (Kirkland *et al.*, 1996). Vollmerhaus *et al.* (2002) reported the change from a diet of soft leaves to a "double diet" of soft leaves and grasses, and eventually to a diet of purely tough fibrous grasses occurred through several phases of Oligocene and Miocene horses (Vollmerhaus *et al.*, 2002). Phylogenetic drift saw the evolution of infundibular enamel cups in incisors and maxillary cheek teeth (CT) resulting in an ever changing occlusal surface with ongoing occlusal dental wear. Vollmerhaus *et al.* propose this results in an equid life-cycle in which the optimal grip of the occlusal surface and efficiency of ingestion favours the young, sexually mature horses, which are at the best age for food intake.

Other dental adaptations to dietary changes included an increase in crown length with prolonged eruption (i.e. they became hypsodont, with reserve crown development), and the presence of cementum peripheral to enamel to allow such prolonged erruption (Bennett, 1992; Kozawa *et al.*, 1988; Mitchell, 2004). Apposition of the three calcified dental tissues (cementum, dentine and enamel) with differential wear rates, allowed CT to 'self-sharpen' during mastication. The harder enamel ridges protruded above the softer dentine and cementum on the occlusal surface (Bennett, 1992; Kilic, 1995). Additionally all the CT (except the first premolar) came into full apposition allowing an even more efficient lateral grinding type of mastication. All these developments have been codified as the branching evolutionary story of the modern horse, *Equus caballus.*

Normal dental wear and the necessity for prophylactic equine dentistry

In his comment on dental wear, Cuddeford explains that "...occlusal wear is a function of three things: the interaction between the two occlusal surfaces [attrition], the time spent chewing and the nature of the material being chewed." (Cuddeford, 2005) To these a fourth could be added - that of the nature of the mineralized dental tissues i.e. whether pathological (e.g. hypoplastic or carious) in nature.

As mentioned in the introduction, the changing climate on Earth during the Oligocene and Miocene Periods and resultant changes in vegetation were the driving force behind the evolution of the equine hypsodont tooth. Different feeding regimes given on a short-term basis to horses may also influence dentition. Studies by Leue (1941) showed that differing feed types changed the degree of lateral excursion of CT during mastication (Leue, 1941). Horses fed concentrates had a greater vertical crushing component in their masticatory cycle with a decreased lateral excursion when compared to those fed hay. Those observed chewing grass were intermediary in lateral jaw excursion.

Diets high in concentrates also greatly limit the length of time horses chew forage and so further predispose to overgrowths from decreased dental attrition (Capper, 1992; Becker, 1962; Capper, 1992; Dixon, 1999). One study looking into the feeding of maize oil as a higher energy replacement for oats reported that such a partial dietary replacement reduced daily NDF by 3% (Lindberg and Karlsson, 2001), thereby reducing to an even greater extent the amount of 'expected' normal dental attrition rather than if the horse had been in its 'natural' environment, grazing the Savannah. Replacing the oats with sugar beet pulp however had the opposite effect, increasing daily NDF by 7%.

Horses fed hay take much longer masticating compared with horses fed a high concentrate/cereal diet (e.g. racehorses in hard work) (Hollands 2004, personal communication; Table 1). One study found horses and ponies to chew hay 58-66 times per minute with 4200 chews /kg DM (Capper, 1992) compared to a second study with horses at grass making 100-105 chewing movements per minute (Myres, 1994). This agrees with Leue's findings of increased lateral excursion (i.e. a slower, longer more deliberate masticatory cycle) being necessary to adequately prepare feed boluses of hay c.f. grass c.f. concentrates.

Table 1. Time required for dietary intake based upon a 500kg horse (Hollands, 2004).

Diet	Time for Mastication
12.5kg forage	16 hours
8kg forage - 4kg concentrates	11.5 hours
3kg forage - 7kg concentrates	6.1 hours

Reduced wear to the occlusal table from decreased time masticating, together with a reduction in degree of lateral excursion of CT when horses are fed a high percentage cereal / concentrate in their diet is the principle reason for the increased formation of sharp dental overgrowths in stabled horses.

Enamel 'points' develop on the buccal occlusal edge of maxillary CT and the lingual occlusal edge of mandibular CT because of uneven occlusal table wear. This arises from:
■ the anisognathic nature of the equine mouth, with mandibular CT being approximately 24% narrower in maxillary CT (Taylor, 2001);
■ differing CT occlusal table widths;
■ the direction and force of the equine masticatory cycle (Tremaine, 1997).

Current advice given by most equine veterinary associations is that routine prophylactic dental procedures should be carried out to remove these enamel points or other focal overgrowths in a regular and timely fashion. In Britain this is usually performed annually or biannually (Dixon *et al.*, 2004). Prophylactic equine dental procedures aim to ensure the mouth is comfortable or at least non-painful when at rest, whilst eating and during exercise.

Reasons given for advocating prophylactic equine dentistry include:
■ To avoid development of dental pathology.
■ To improve control of the head when being ridden or driven.
■ To improve feed digestibility.

Although discussion of these first two points is not the topic of this paper, it is important to remember that dental disorders are of major clinical importance in the horse. A recent abattoir survey in Britain showed that 72% of the skulls examined had dental abnormalities that would have benefited from dental treatment (Brigham and Duncanson, 2000). In the USA equine dental disorders were ranked as the third most common medical problem encountered by large animal practitioners (Traub-Dargatz *et al.*, 1991). One survey found that 24% of young horses in the USA without clinical signs of dental disease had dental abnormalities and suggested that proper dental examinations were often neglected because of the perceived dangers and difficulties associated with such examinations (Uhlinger, 1987). Another found that over 80%

of 500 skulls examined showed evidence of oral disease or dental pathology (Kirkland *et al.*, 1994). Dixon *et al.* (2000) noted horses with disorders of wear exhibited the highest incidence (70%) of quidding (the dropping of feed during masticatory movements) of all dental diseases (Dixon *et al.*, 2000a). Clinical evidence shows contemporary dental procedures can correct most types of dental pathology present and delay reoccurrence of dental overgrowths (Dixon *et al.*, 2000a; Dixon *et al.*, 2000b; Dixon *et al.*, 1999a).

Dentistry to improve feed digestibility

In one of the few studies to determine if current prophylactic equine dental procedures had an effect on feed digestibility in horses, Ralston *et al.* (2001) looked at whether performing routine dental correction (removal of enamel points or focal overgrowths from CT) improved digestion of a hay / grain ration; compared with CT that had received a 'performance' float (rounding and smoothing of the dental arcades, including the occlusal surface) (Ralston *et al.*, 2001). They found that apparent digestibility of crude protein and fibre was reduced if the occlusal angle of CT 307 (3rd left mandibular premolar) was greater than 80 degrees relative to the vertical axis i.e. the CT had been 'flattened' excessively when under-going a performance float. Routine correction of small enamel overgrowths did not improve feed digestibility in this study. This was also observed in a later study by Carmalt who suggested that dental floating did not result in significant short-term changes in body weight, body condition score, feed digestibility, or faecal particle size in healthy pregnant mares (Carmalt *et al.*, 2004).

As mentioned previously however, regular floating of sharp enamel points and hooks can prevent their progression to causing more serious oral pathology such as oral ulceration, periodontal disease, major dental overgrowths and conditions such as shear-mouth (Dixon *et al.*, 2000a; Dacre, 2004a; Scrutchfield, 1999). Low body condition score has been linked to presence of dental pathology in a study of 300 debilitated working equids (100 horses, 100 donkeys and 100 mules) (Roy, 2002). Forty-seven percent of horses, 32% of donkeys and 80% of mules with a body condition score of one or less had significant dental pathology present.

Dietary influence on dental development and acquired pathological conditions

In addition to the actions of domestication potentially reducing overall dental wear and the consequent formation of sharp dental overgrowths, diet may also contribute to more specific dental pathology.

Odontodystrophies are diseases of teeth caused by nutritional, metabolic and toxic insults. The most obvious effects of osteodystrophies appear in enamel, as once formed, enamel is not able to be repaired following the subsequent apoptosis of the ameloblast cells that formed it. Enamel lesions however are less evident in equine teeth that have a layer of cementum lying over most of the enamel present in clinical crown (c.f. brachydont teeth). Depending on the severity of nutritional deficiency, ameloblasts may produce no enamel, a little enamel, or poorly mineralised enamel (Barker *et al.*, 1993). Defects affect all teeth currently forming enamel and will usually be bilaterally symmetrical when of nutritional origin.

Odontoblasts (dentine progenitor cells) and cementoblasts (cementum progenitor cells) are also susceptible to nutritional or other physiological insults; however they may be replenished from undifferentiated cells of the dental pulp or periodontal ligament. Thus lesions in actively forming dentine or cementum may be repaired, whereas those in enamel are permanent. Although a nutritional link has not been specifically made to horses, dental hypoplasia has been observed in all three calcified dental tissues, as has globular dentine - an indication of dentine hypomineralisation (Baker, 1979a; Dacre, 2004b).

The progressive attrition of equine teeth necessitates the continued deposition of secondary dentine to prevent pulp exposure. This metabolically demanding process requires a significant blood supply (with appropriate levels of transported minerals) to the dentinogenic zone of the pulp cavity, which must be prolonged well into a horse's life (Dixon and Copeland, 1993). A similarly rich vascular supply is present for the continued formation of peripheral cementum (Mitchell, 2004). Teeth formed during periods of hypocalcaemia are very susceptible to wear, to the point of exposing dental pulp. This has been reported in sheep and has been suspected as being one of the aetiologies of apical infection in horses (Dixon *et al.*, 2000b; Thurley,

1985). Calcium deficiency has also been associated with delayed eruption of teeth.

A study by Engstrom and Noren (1986) observed that maxillary incisors of young rats fed a diet deficient in calcium and vitamin D for four weeks developed hypoplastic enamel surfaces. In this dietary regime nutritional secondary hyperparathyroidism resulted. The plasma parameters returned to normal within the experiment's timeframe and were maintained, but only at the expense of progressive bone loss. The calcium loss from bone was generalized but the bones were not uniformly affected, with loss being greatest from the jaw bones, especially alveolar bone. Loss of alveolar bone has been linked as an initiating factor in periodontal disease in animals (Krook *et al.*, 1975). Osseous lesions in animal nutritional secondary hyperparathyroidism are reversible by correction of dietary calcium and phosphorus levels, provided osteodystrophic fibrosis has not developed. Limited experiments in human periodontal disease indicate that added dietary calcium can positively influence the alveolar bone loss (Krook *et al.*, 1972).

In 1906 Colyer described periodontal disease as the 'scourge of the horse,' finding this disease present in approximately one third of 484 skulls examined (Miles and Grigson, 1990). Baker (1970) recorded an incidence of 60% periodontal disease in horses aged over 15 years (Baker, 1979b) and later Wafa (1988) reported an overall incidence of 37% of periodontal disease in the abattoir specimens examined, with 52% of animals showing concurrent periodontitis as their teeth were erupting (Wafa, 1988). Again the disease was more prevalent in older animals, reaching a peak of 60% in horses over 20 years of age.

Primary equine periodontal disease however is uncommon (Dixon, 1992). Dixon found only 7% of cases referred with incisor dental problems to be affected by primary periodontitis and 4% in referred mandibular and maxillary CT cases (Dixon *et al.*, 1999a; Dixon, 1992). The higher incidences described in previous studies may be due to the inclusion of periodontal disease arising secondarily from other primary pathology such as displaced teeth. It is interesting to note however that periodontal disease increased with age, where chronic alveolar bone loss may have arisen from inadequate calcium intake in some cases and therefore had some interaction with development of periodontal disease.

Diet has been more directly implicated in the aetiology of equine periodontal disease. Hofmeyer (1960) attributed a diet of coarse or chopped food as a predisposing factor to periodontal disease in South African horses, where he claimed this to be of major importance (Hofmeyer, 1960). In contrast to most other reports, he stated that the maxillary CT rows were more commonly affected with periodontitis than mandibular CT rows. Feeding of chaff, where small pieces of food can become impacted between teeth, is thought to initiate gingival damage either mechanically or through bacterial fermentation of these foodstuffs (Miles and Grigson, 1990).

Food impaction in the interdental space with associated periodontal disease has been treated by the employment of two techniques. The first aims at widening the interdental space, thus allowing food to pass freely between the teeth, no longer becoming trapped and developing associated destruction of the periodontium (Dixon *et al.*, 1999b; Carmalt, 2003). The second involves the cleaning out, debriding and packing of such periodontal pockets (perioceutic therapy) in conjunction with correction of any associated dental malocclusion (Klugh, 2005).

Periodontal disease is now ranked as the most significant dental condition in man, with 50% of adults aged 55-64 years in one survey having severe (>4mm periodontal attachment loss) periodontal disease (National Institute of Dental and Craniofacial Research, 2003). The lower prevalence of periodontal disease in 'lower animals' is cited as one reason why research in this area of human medicine has been relatively unsuccessful to date (Shafer *et al.*, 1983).

Caries

Historically the most notorious association between diet and dental conditions was that of caries formation. The role of diet in the aetiology of caries has remained largely unchanged since first postulated by Miller in 1889. Miller's acidogenic theory proposed acid from the fermentation of dietary carbohydrates by oral bacteria, led to progressive decalcification of tooth substance with subsequent destruction of the organic matrix. More recent work has shown that when dietary sugars are metabolised by bacteria to lactic acid, plaque pH will fall, for example by two units within 10 minutes of sugar ingestion by humans

(Critchley *et al.*, 1967). When plaque pH reaches 5.5 or below, mineral ions are released from calcium hydroxyapatite crystals (which make up the vast majority of mineralised dental tissue substance), and then diffuse into the adjacent plaque, and thereafter the oral cavity where they are lost from the oral micro-environment (Soames and Southam, 1993). Such mineral loss principally occurs from teeth during prolonged acidic attacks.

Promotion of sound dietary practices is an integral part of contemporary caries management in humans (Mobley, 2003). The following principles are now advised by human dental health professionals to encourage good oral health and decrease caries risk:

- "Encourage balanced diets based on moderation and variety as depicted by the Food Guide Pyramid. Avoid references to "bad" foods and focus on "good" diets that include a variety of foods.
- Give examples of how combining and sequencing foods can enhance mastication, saliva production, and oral clearance at each eating occasion. Combining dairy foods with sugary foods, raw foods with cooked, and protein-rich foods with acidogenic foods are all good examples. Suggest that eating and drinking be followed by cariostatic foods such as xylitol chewing gum.
- Drink water to satisfy thirst and hydration needs as often as possible. Restrict consumption of sweetened beverages to meal and snack times when they can be combined with other cariostatic foods.
- When a patient reports excessive dietary intake of a fermentable carbohydrate to the point of displacing other important foods in the diet, identify alternatives that will help the patient maintain or achieve a healthy body weight, oral health status, and a nutrient-dense intake".

Human data suggests a lifelong synergy between nutrition and the integrity of the oral cavity in health and disease (Touger-Decker and Mobley, 2003).

Caries of cementum, enamel and dentine have been identified in the horse, most frequently in cementum - this being both the softest, least mineralised calcified dental tissue, and being the most prevalent (with respect to surface area exposure) in the equine oral cavity (Dacre, 2004b). Early studies reported incidences of infundibular caries to be as high as 79-100% in certain ages of equine populations (Baker, 1970;

Honma *et al.*, 1962). More recently infundibular caries was reported to occur in 12% of maxillary CT, but not in incisors (0%) (Dixon *et al.*, 2000a; Dixon *et al.*, 1999a). Infundibular caries appears grossly as a darkly stained region within the infundibular cemental lakes (Kilic *et al.*, 1997). This dark staining may potentially extend beyond the infundibular cementum into both the enamel and adjacent dentine. The presence of food within equine hypoplastic infundibular cementum can promote infundibular caries which, depending on bacteria present, amount and type of food present, and time has been proposed as another potential aetiology for apical infection (Baker, 1974; Schumacher and Honnas, 1993).

The pathological significance of peripheral cemental caries is unknown however, by weakening and removing occlusal cementum (that contributes considerably to equine CT clinical crown structure) (Mitchell, 2004), it may both increase the rate of occlusal wear and contribute to the development of diastema and associated periodontal disease. Removal of peripheral cementum also makes proud areas of brittle enamel on the occlusal surface more prone to fracture.

Dentition and the influence of diet selection

There has been no work in horses on the role the state of dentition may play in diet selection. This however has become a field in its own right in humans, particularly when considering the elderly where dental state is usually compromised. A strong link has been shown between dietary variety, nutrient intake and oral health. Chewing ability in humans is highly correlated with the number of teeth present, but the relationship is not linear (Sheiham and Steele, 2001). People who cannot chew or bite comfortably are less likely to consume high-fibre foods such as bread, fruit and vegetables thereby reducing their intake of essential nutrients (Brodeur *et al.*, 1993). Mean daily nutrient intake has been shown to be statistically lower in subjects who had fewer teeth or ill-fitting dentures than in subjects who had more natural/functional teeth (Marshall *et al.*, 2002; Laurin, D. *et al.*, 1992). In one study of 1755 people aged over 65 years, 13% with impaired dentition said that they 'often' or 'always' had problems chewing or biting, with one in five reporting that oral conditions prevented them from eating foods they would choose and that 15% took longer to complete their meal (Atchison and Dolan, 1990).

Articles written on appropriate dental care for geriatric horses often focus on not raising the expectations of the owner to being able to achieve a completely '100% successful result', and that attention to dietary modification should be encouraged (Lowder and Mueller, 1998). The potential for further development of dietary alternatives for the aging equine populations of the developed world are still largely un-tapped, and likely to be an area of growth in the coming years.

Conclusions

"The animal [horse] *was sent on this earth provided with every apparatus necessary to crop, to comminute, and to digest the green verdure of the earth...To fit the creature for his uses, he changes the character of its food. Artificially-prepared oats and hay, with various condiments, are used to stimulate the spirit. No one enquires whether such a diet is the fitting support of the animal? But, when the energy lags, beans, beer, &c., &c., are resorted to as restoratives for exhaustion. The quadruped, thus treated, men have agreed shall be aged by the eighth year."* Mayhew (1873).

In the above statement Mayhew is adamant that incorrect diet will lead to premature aging of horses, and later goes even further to state this may lead to their death. In his opening statement he is equally adamant that these same animals are perfectly suited to their natural environment and staple diet of eating "the green verdure." Luckily our knowledge of equine nutrition has come a long way since the feeding of 'beer and beans' as restoratives in 1873. But that is not to say that supplement based diets have overcome all obstacles so forcefully attacked by Mayhew.

Equine dentistry has undertaken a renaissance during the past 15 years as evidenced by the publication of at least five textbooks solely on this topic during this same period where previously there were none. It can be expected that owner's knowledge of equine dentistry will follow the professions. With increasing owner vigilance, practitioner knowledge and skill at diagnosis and treatment, and continued academic research in this field, many of the relationships found to exist between diet, the health status of the oral cavity and dentistry in humans and other species may be equally true for equids.

Ian Dacre

References

Atchison, K.A. and Dolan, T.A., 1990. Development of the Geriatric Oral Health Assessment Index. J. Dent. Educ. 54, p. 680-687.

Baker, G.J., 1970. Some aspects of equine dental disease. Equine Vet. J. 2, p. 105-110.

Baker, G.J., 1974. Some aspects of equine dental decay. Equine Vet. J. 6, p. 127-130.

Baker, G.J., 1979a. A study of dental disease in the horse. 1-96. 1979. Glasgow University.

Baker, G.J., 1979b. Dental disease in horses. In Practice 19-26.

Barker, I.K., Van Dreumel, A.A. and Palmer, 1993. N. Pathology of Domestic Animals. Jubb,K.V.F., Kennedy,P.C. & Palmer,N. (eds.), Academic Press, San Diego. pp. 1-33

Becker, E. , 1962. Zahne. Verlag Paul Parey, Berlin.

Bennett, D., 1992. Horse Breeding and Management. Evans,J.W. (ed.), Elsevier, Amsterdam, , pp. 1-37.

Brigham, E.J. and Duncanson, G., 2000. An equine postmortem study: 50 cases. Equine Vet Edu 12, p. 59-62.

Brodeur, J.M., Laurin, D., Vallee, R. and Lachapelle, D., 1993. Nutrient intake and gastrointestinal disorders related to masticatory performance in the edentulous elderly. J. Prosthet. Dent. 70, p. 468-473.

Budiansky, S., 1997. The nature of horses: their evolution, intelligence and behaviour. Weidenfield & Nicolson, London.

Capper, S.R. 1992. The effects of feed types on ingestive behaviour in different horse types. P.1-160. University of Edinburgh.

Carmalt, J.L., 2003. Understanding the equine diastema. Equine Vet Edu 15, p. 34-35.

Carmalt, J.L., Townsend, H.G., Janzen, E.D. and Cymbaluk, N.E., 2004. Effect of dental floating on weight gain, body condition score, feed digestibility, and fecal particle size in pregnant mares. J. Am. Vet. Med. Assoc. 225, p. 1889-1893.

Critchley, P., Wood, J.M., Saxton, C.A. and Leach, S.A., 1967. The polymerisation of dietary sugars by dental plaque. Caries Res. 1, p. 112-129.

Cuddeford, D., 2005. Feeding, management and equine dentistry. Vet. Rec. 156, p. 751.

Dacre, I.T., 2004a. Equine Dentistry. Baker G.J.and Easley J. (ed.), Elsevier, London.

Dacre, I.T., 2004b. A Pathological, Histological and Ultrastructural Study of Diseased Equine Teeth. Royal (Dick) School for Veterinary Studies.

Dixon, P.M. and Copeland, A.N., 1993. The radiological appearance of mandibular cheek teeth in ponies of different ages. Equine Vet Edu 5, p. 317-323.

Dixon, P.M. *et al.*, 1999a Equine dental disease part 1: a long-term study of 400 cases: disorders of incisor, canine and first premolar teeth. Equine Vet. J. 31, p. 369-377.

Dixon, P.M. *et al.*, 1999b. Equine dental disease part 2: a long-term study of 400 cases: disorders of development and eruption and variations in position of the cheek teeth. Equine Vet. J. 31, p. 519-528.

Dixon, P.M. *et al.*, 2000a. Equine dental disease. Part 3: A long-term study of 400 cases: disorders of wear, traumatic damage and idiopathic fractures, tumours and miscellaneous disorders of the cheek teeth. Equine Vet. J. 32, p. 9-18.

Dixon, P.M. *et al.*, 2000b Equine dental disease part 4: a long-term study of 400 cases: apical infections of cheek teeth. Equine Vet. J. 32, p.182-194.

Dixon, P.M. *et al.*, 2004. Survey of the provision of prophylactic dental care for horses in Great Britain and Ireland between 1999 and 2002. Vet. Rec. 155, p. 693-698.

Dixon, P.M., 1992. Equine cheek tooth disease - is periodontal disease still a problem? p. 1-8. 4-2-1992.

Dixon, P.M., 1999. Equine Dentistry. Baker G.J.and Easley J. (ed.), W.B. Saunders, London, pp. 3-28.

Engstrom, C. and Noren, J.G., 1986. Effects of orthodontic force on enamel formation in normal and hypocalcemic rats. J. Oral Pathol. 15, 78-82.

Hofmeyer, C.F.B., 1960. Comparitive dental pathology. J. South African Veterinary Medical Association 29, p.471-480.

Honma, K., Yamakawa, M., Yamauchi, S. and Hosoya, S., 1962. Statistical study on the occurrence of dental caries of domestic animals. Jap. J. Vet. Res. 10, p. 31-37.

Kilic, S., 1995. A light and electron microscopic study of calcified dental tissues in normal horses. p.. 1-193. University of Edinburgh. Ref Type: Thesis/Dissertation

Kilic, S., Dixon, P.M. and Kempson, S.A., 1997. A light microscopic and ultrastructural examination of calcified dental tissues on horses: 4. Cement and the amelocemental junction [see comments]. Equine Vet. J. 29, p. 213-219.

Kirkland, K.D., Baker, G.J., Marretta, S., Eurell, J.A. and Losonsky, J.M., 1996. Effects of aging on the endodontic system, reserve crown, and roots of equine mandibular cheek teeth. Am. J. Vet. Res. 57, 31-38.

Kirkland, K.D., Maretta, S.M., Inoue, O.J. and Baker, G.J., 1994. Survey of equine dental disease and associated oral pathology. (40), Proc. Am. Ass. equine Practnrs. p. 119-120.

Klugh, D.O., 2005. Treatment of Equine Periodontal Disease. 30-34. University of Minnesota. Ref Type: Conference Proceeding

Kozawa, Y., Mishima, H. and Sakae, T., 1988. Evolution of tooth structure in the Equoidea. J. Nihon Univ Sch Dent. 30, p. 287-296.

Krook, L., Whalen, J.P., Lesser, G.V. and Berens, D.L., 1975. Experimental studies on osteoporosis. Methods Achiev. Exp. Pathol. 7, p. 72-108.

Krook, L., Whalen, J.P., Lesser, G.V. and Lutwak, L., 1972. Human periodontal disease and osteoporosis. Cornell Vet. 62, p.371-391.

Laurin, D. *et al.*, 1992. Nutritional deficiencies and gastrointestinal disorders in the edentulous elderly: a literature review. J. Can. Dent. Assoc. 58, p. 738-740.

Leue, G., 1941. Handbuch der speziellen pathologischen anatomie der haustiere. J. Dobberstein, G.P.a.H.S. (ed.), Verlag Paul Parey, Berlin, pp. 131-132

Lindberg, J.E. and Karlsson, C.P., 2001 Effect of partial replacement of oats with sugar beet pulp and maize oil on nutrient utilisation in horses. Equine Vet. J. 33, p. 585-590.

Lowder, M.Q. and Mueller, P.O., 1998. Dental disease in geriatric horses. Vet. Clin. North Am. Equine Pract. 14, p. 365-380.

Marshall, T.A., Warren, J.J., Hand, J.S., Xie, X.J. and Stumbo, P.J., 2002. Oral health, nutrient intake and dietary quality in the very old. J. Am. Dent. Assoc. 133, p. 1369-1379.

Mayhew, E., 1873. The Illustrated Horse Management., W.H. Allen, London pp. 135-175.

Miles, A.E.W. and Grigson, C., 1990. Colyer's Variations and diseases of the teeth of animals. Cambridge University Press, Cambridge.

Miller, W.D., 1889. Die mikroorganismen des mundhohle. Leipzig.

Mitchell, S., 2004. Peripheral cementum of normal equine cheek teeth: a qualitative and quantitative study. p. 1-146. University of Edinburgh.

Mobley, C.C., 2003. Nutrition and dental caries. Dent. Clin. North Am. 47, p. 319-336.

Myres, J.S., 1994. The effects of boby size, grass height and time of day on the foraging behaviour of horses. 56. Aberystwyth University. Ref Type: Thesis/Dissertation

National Institute of Dental and Craniofacial Research, 2003. Periodontal diseases: microbial and host genomics / proteomics. 4-24-2003. Ref Type: Internet Communication

Ralston, S.L., Foster, D.L., Divers, T. and Hintz, H.F., 2001. Effect of dental correction on feed digestibility in horses. Equine Vet. J. 33, p. 390-393.

Roy, C. 2002. Dental problems in debilitated equines in Delhi. p. 267-270. Hama, Syria. Proceedings of the Fourth International Colloquiem on Working Equines. 4-20-2002.

Schumacher, J. and Honnas, C.M., 1993. Dental Surgery. Vet. Clin. North Am. Equine Pract. 9, p. 133-152.

Scrutchfield, W.L., 1999 Equine Dentistry. Baker,G.J. & Easley,J. (eds.), W.B.Saunders Co. Ltd., London, pp. 185-205.

Shafer, W.G., Hine, M.K. and Levy, B.M., 1983 A textbook of oral pathology., W.B.Saunders Company, Philadelphia, pp. 760-805.

Sheiham, A. and Steele, J., 2001. Does the condition of the mouth and teeth affect the ability to eat certain foods, nutrient and dietary intake and nutritional status amongst older people? Public Health Nutr. 4, p. 797-803.

Soames, J.V. and Southam, J.C., 1993. Oral Pathology. Soames,J.V. & Southam,J.C. (eds.), Oxford University Press, Oxford, pp. 19-33.

Taylor, A.C., 2001. An investigation of mandibular width and related dental disorders in the equine oral cavity. Coventry University. Ref Type: Thesis/Dissertation

Thurley, D.C., 1985. The pathogenesis of ecxcessive wear in permanent teeth of sheep. New Zealand Veterinary Journal 33, p.24-26.

Touger-Decker, R. and Mobley, C.C., 2003. Position of the American Dietetic Association: Oral health and nutrition. J. Am. Diet. Assoc. 103, p. 615-625.

Traub-Dargatz, J.L., Salman, M.D. and Voss, J.L., 1991. Medical problems of adult horses, as ranked by equine practitioners. J. Am. Vet Med. Assoc. 198, p. 1745-1747.

Tremaine, W.H., 1997. Dental care in horses. In Practice 19, p. 186-199.

Uhlinger, C., 1987. Survey of selected dental abnormalities in 233 horses. 33, Proceedings of the 33rd Annual Convention of the Association of Equine Practitioners. p. 577-583.

Vollmerhaus,B., Roos,H. and Knospe,C., 2002. The origin and function of the enamel cup, infundibulum dentis, on the incisors of the horse. Anat. Histol. Embryol. 31, p. 53-59.

Wafa, N.S., 1988. A study of dental disease in the horse. 1-205. National University of Ireland, Faculty of Veterinary Medicine, University College Dublin.

Nutritional management to keep the hoof healthy

Hans Geyer
Veterinär-Anatomisches Institut, Universität Zürich

Introduction

The nutritional influence on hoof horn quality is only one part of the various influences, which are frequently overestimated. People hope that they can solve all problems as cracks, white line diseases, thin soles or thrush by adding a supplement to the food. First of all we have to think about the different influences to hoof horn quality and the anatomical-physiological basis for the production of a sound horn with a high loading capacity. After these reflections we will inform about some encouraging results where nutrition or nutritional supplements were able to improve the hoof conditions that they were in a healthy or a better condition than before.

The different influences on the hoof should be kept in mind:
- Genetical influences on horn production, horn quality and the hoof form.
- Nutritional influences in horn production and its hoof horn quality.
- Environmental influences:
  - humidity, temperature, feces and urine in beddings;
  - work of the horse and quality of the soil;
  - hoof care and farriery.

At the beginning some anatomical basics shall be mentioned, which are necessary to understand the possibilities and the limits of the different influences. Some information about weak points in the construction shall be given as well. Concerning nutritional influences we will focus to those factors where experiences from own trials are present.

The hoof (Figure 1) consists of central stabilizing parts as bones, ligaments, tendons and the surrounding modified skin. This modified

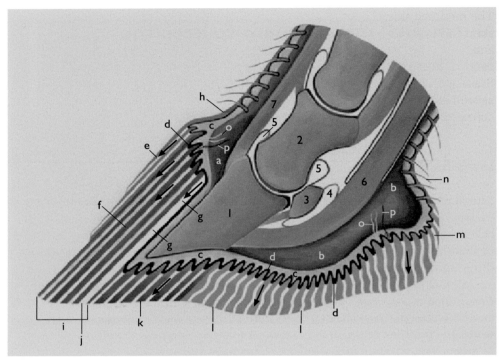

Figure 1. Schematic longitudinal section of a horses hoof.
1. coffin bone; 2. short pastern, middle phalanx; 3. navicular bone; 4. navicular bursa;
5. coffin joint; 6. deep flexor tendon; 7. extensor tendon.
a. subcutis of coronary band; b. subcutis of the frog and heel; c. dermis = corium
with papillae; d. epidermis, germinative layer; e. perioplic horn; f. coronary horn;
g. horn leaflets; h. coronary border; i. bearing border; j. white line; k. sole horn; l. frog
horn; m. heel horn; n. hairy skin; o. blood vessels; p. nerves.
The bright lines symbolize horn tubules
arrows = direction of growth

skin is hairless and has enormous keratinized layers. In these keratinized layers the horn cells are not only superposed (one above the other) but they are arranged in most parts as tubules to get a very high stability with a relative low portion of material (Bolliger and Geyer, 1992). The horn cells, which are dead, have to hold together over several months and in the horn wall more than one year, before they may be rubbed off at the different surfaces.

The modified skin of the hoof consists of the same layers as the hairy skin: the subcutis and the cutis. The subcutis has cushioning effects and is only present in areas, where cushioning is desired: at the coronary band, in the frog and the heels. The subcutis is made of connective tissue with blood vessels and nerves and contains sometimes fat cells as well. The cutis has two parts, the corium or dermis, consisting of connective tissue and the epidermis, which is avascular.

The dermis has to nourish the epidermis and has to bring all feedstuffs to the epidermis which are used for the production of sound and resistant epidermal cells. The second task of the dermis = corium should make a mechanical firm connection to the epidermis. For both, nutrition and the mechanical tight connection a large surface of the corium is necessary. This large surface is realized in form of high papillae or in form of leaflets, which are visible with naked eye, because they are some millimeters high.

The epidermis, consisting of epithelial cells, has in the basal area the germinative layer of live cells with its stratum basale, the main area of cell-division, and the following stratum spinosum of many cell layers. In zones with hard keratin the stratum corneum (e.g. coronary horn) succeeds immediately after the stratum spinosum. In areas with soft keratin (e.g. the periople, hairy skin) a stratum granulosum, which contains keratohyaline granula, is interposed between stratum spinosum and stratum corneum. In the stratum corneum the epithelial cells are dead but they frequently contain pycnotic, shrunken nuclei.

The inner cohesive strength filaments are synthesized in the stratum basale and spinosum. The filaments, which are proteins come together to form bundles already in the stratum spinosum. The cohesion between the epithelial cells is formed by desmosomes in the stratum basale and spinosum, but of an intercellular glue or intercellular cement in the stratum corneum (Figures 2, 3). This intercellular glue is mainly responsible for the strength and the quality of the horn. The intercellular glue is synthesized in the stratum spinosum in form of granules which are given in the intercellular space near the stratum corneum. The intercellular glue consists to a great part of glycoproteins, which stain red because of its carbohydrates with the histochemical Periodic-Acid-Schiff reaction (= PAS reaction). The good cohesion of the horn cells

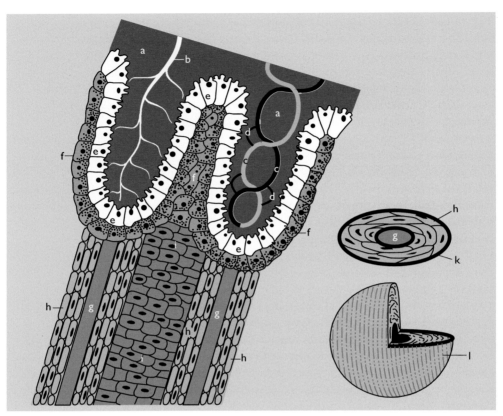

Figure 2. Detail of dermal papillae and epidermis in the external zone of the coronary segment.
a. corium; b. nerve; c. blood vessels; d. capillaries; e-l. epidermis: e. stratum basale; f. stratum spinosum with desmosomes - the granules are precursors of the intercellular glue, which is present between the cell membranes of the stratum corneum; g-l: stratum corneum: g-h: horn tubules, g. marrow; h. cortex; i. intertubular horn; k. transverse section of an oval tubule; l. flat horn cells in a pancake form.

can be estimated by measuring the tensile strength of hoof horn under standardized conditions.

It must be pointed out that hoof horn strength may only be changed or improved, if factors and especially nutritional factors are influencing the germinative layer of the epidermis. In the transformation of keratins from soft to hard keratine cysteine is transformed to cystine with the

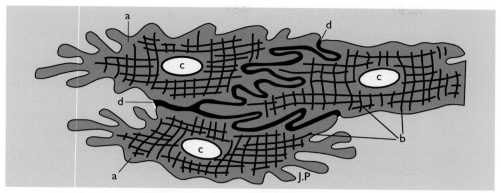

Figure 3. Flat horn cells and their intercellular connections.
a. keratin cells with interdigitations at the sharp end of the cells; b. keratin fibers in different directions; c. pycnotic nuclei; d. intercellular glue.

double S-S bonding. The sulfur-containing amino acids methionine and cystine are important nutrients for the keratin-synthesis. But the right "program" for these synthesis, occurring mainly in the ribosomes, is also genetically fixed and small changes in this program may result in early decaying horn cells. It should always be remembered that it takes several months after the horn production until improvements or damage in the horn will be seen in the superficial or distal layers of the horn shoe.

In most areas of the hoof the horn is produced in form of tubules (Figure 2). Distal to the dermal papillae the germinative layer of the epidermis produces the horn tubules. At the tip of the papillae the epidermal cells soon decay as a form of programmed cell death. This central part of the tubule with decayed cells forms the tubular marrow. At the side part of the papillae the epidermis produces the cortical cells, flat or spindle shaped cells, which have to be very resistant and form the tubular cortex. The tubular cortex is the most important weight bearing structure of the hoof horn. Between the papillae the germinative epidermal layer produces the intertubular horn where the cells are less regularly arranged. In horses a slight border can be seen between the tubular cortex and the intertubular horn.

The hoof has certain properties in its different parts, not only in the hoof horn but also in the corium and in the subcutis (Figure 1).

Therefore the hoof is divided in regions or segments: perioplic-, coronary-, wall segment; sole-, frog- and heel segment. Each segment consists of epidermis, corium, and, if cushioning is desired, also of a subcutis. The corium and subcutis are very sensitive. The nerve endings reach the dermal papillae and in maximum the deep layers of the epidermis. The stratum corneum is not sensitive. Pain is only induced if the thin germinative layer and the corium or the subcutis are irritated.

The horn wall, which contains horn of the three dorsal and lateral segments, has a proximal borderline to the hairy skin, which is named coronary border. The distal border of the horn wall, which bears to a certain amount the body weight, is named weight bearing border or bearing border.

Dorsal and lateral in the hooves we find proximally the perioplic segment, with a soft and sometimes fissured horn which covers and protects the underlying coronary horn. The perioplic horn is regularly seen in the proximal part of the horn wall. In unshod horses it may reach the bearing border. In horses with shoes the distal part of the perioplic horn is regularly rasped off.

The coronary segment produces a hard and very resistant horn, which is the most important part of the horn wall and is about 10 mm thick in the anterior part of the horn wall. The coronary horn can be divided in an external, middle and inner zone (Figure 4). In the external and middle zone tubules with flat cortical cells and oval diameter are found, whereas in the inner zone a different type of tubules with round diameter and spindle shaped cortical cells is present. The wall segment, which begins approx. 2 cm distal of the coronary border (Figure 1), contains soft leaflets, which consist of corium and the covering germinative layer of the epidermis (Figures 4-5). Between the soft leaflets the very thin horn leaflets are found. The horn leaflets are produced from the germinative layer at the transition of the coronary to the wall segment. Both the horn leaflets and the soft leaflets must be very well connected because at this connection the inner parts of the hooves are fixed to the horn wall.

The horn wall is composed of horn of all segments perioplic horn, coronary horn and horn leaflets (Figures 1, 4, 6, 7). The coronary horn is the largest and the most important part of it. In the lateral and

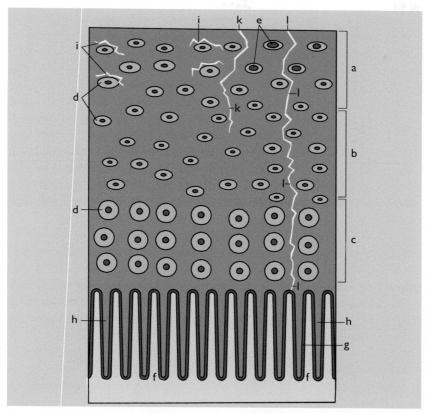

Figure 4. Transverse section through the middle part of the horn wall with leaflets of the wall segment and some pathological changes.
a-c. coronary horn: a. external; b. middle; c. inner zone; d. normal tubules; e. tubules with enlarged marrows; f-g. soft leaflets: f. dermis; g. germinative layer of epidermis (dark); h. horn leaflets; i. micro-cracks in the external zone; k. superficial crack; l. deep crack, which often induces pain.

palmar/plantar direction, the horn wall gets thinner, a condition which allows the lateral extension of the quarters in the hoof mechanism. But in some animals the horn wall is too thin in the quarters, because the coronary band is too small and the thin quarters are predisposed to cracks (Figure 7). The coronary horn and the horn leaflets are palmar/plantar inflexed as bars, which run parallel to the frog and normally prevent a too wide lateral extension of the quarters (Figure 7).

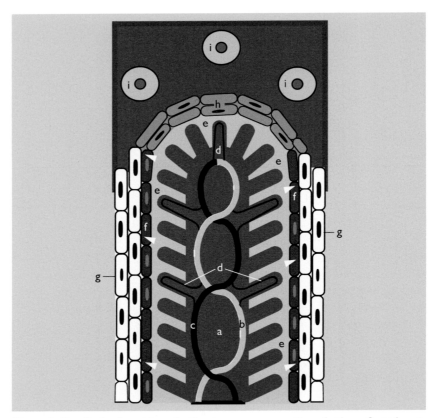

Figure 5. Detail of soft and horn leaflets in transverse sections. In the soft epidermis (e) damage and detachment occurs in laminitis.
a. dermis = corium; b-d. blood vessels: b. arteriole; c. venole; d. capillaries; e. stratum germinativum of epidermis; f. small horn cells growing horizontally and connecting the big horn cells (g), which grow in proximo-distal direction; h. cap horn; i. tubules of the inner zone of coronary horn.

In the coronary horn some weak points appear: already in the proximal parts, in the outer zone of the coronary horn, cracks are frequently seen at the border between cortex and intertubular horn (Figure 4). Occasionally some tubules with enlarged marrows can be found which develop from premature decay of inner cortical cells. In the distal horn wall, near the bearing border, many micro-cracks appear between the middle and inner zone of the coronary horn - a weak point where the two different types of tubules come together (Figure 6). Hoof nails should not be placed in this area, but if possible, in the white line.

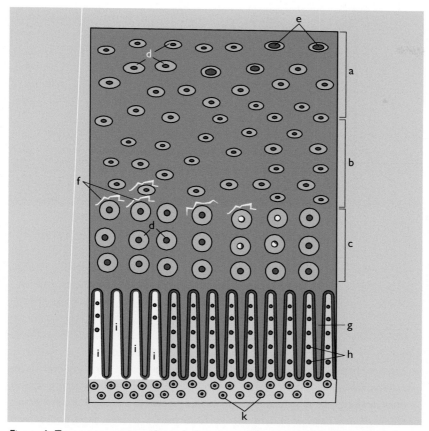

Figure 6. Transverse sections through the coronary horn and white line at the bearing border (Munzinger, 2005).

a-c. coronary horn: a external zone; b. middle zone; c. inner zone; d. normal tubules; e. tubules with enlarged marrows; f. micro-cracks which are frequently found between the middle and inner zone of the coronary horn; g-i. white line: g. horn leaflets; h. terminal horn = tubular horn; i. hollow spaces, where terminal horn is detached from the horn leaflets - in soft white lines; k. sole horn.

Cracks in the hoof horn frequently are seen parallel to the horn tubules and rarely transverse to the tubules. The cracks do not cause pain if they are superficial; if they reach in depth near to the dermis they often are painful (Figure 4, 8).

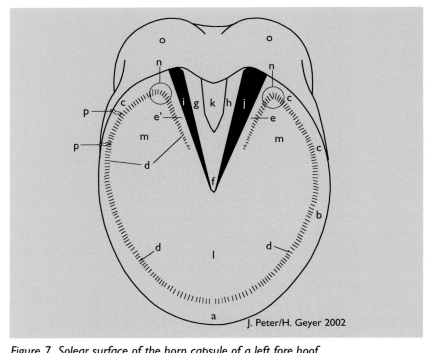

Figure 7. Solear surface of the horn capsule of a left fore hoof.
a. coronary horn, dorsal part; b. coronary horn, lateral part; c. coronary horn in the
quarter; d. white line; e medial bar, e' lateral bar; f-h. frog: f. tip of the frog; g. lateral,
h. medial ridge of the frog; i-j. lateral and medial grooves of the frog; k. central groove
of the frog; l. sole anterior part; m. sole posterior part; n. palmar angle; o. heel horn;
p. cracks in the thin wall of the lateral quarter.

In the distal part of the wall segment the soft leaflets may not appear at the bearing border. Otherwise each step would be painful. Therefore the soft leaflets split into papillae beginning approx. 2 cm proximal to the bearing border (Figure 1). The adjacent epidermis which covers this papillae produces again a tubular horn which fills as terminal horn the space between the horn leaflets (Figure 6). Both, the horn leaflets and the terminal horn form the white line (Figures 6, 7), which connects the horn wall with the sole. Very often the terminal horn decays and detaches from the horn leaflets, resulting in the smeary, weak white lines, today also named as "white line disease" (Figures 6, 9).

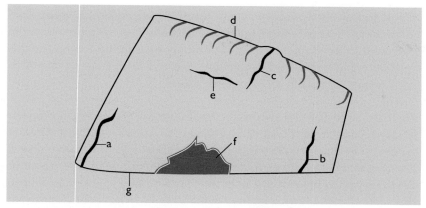

Figure 8. Lateral view of a hoof with hoof horn changes.
a. longitudinal crack = sand crack at the toe; b. sand crack at the quarter; c. proximal crack which comes from the coronary border (d); e. transverse crack; f. broken-out area near the bearing border (g).

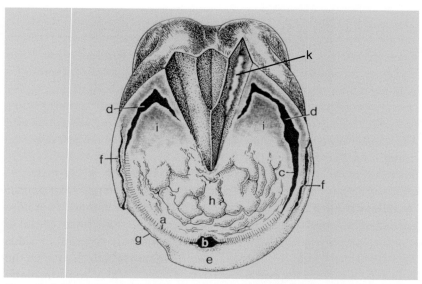

Figure 9. Solear surface of a fore hoof with pathological changes (Josseck et al., 1995).
a. normal white line; b-d. soft parts of the white line: b. at the toe; c. at the medial part; d. in the quarters of the bearing border; e. normal coronary horn at the toe; f. cracks in the lateral and medial part of coronary horn; g. broken out part of coronary horn; h. crumbly horn in the anterior part of the sole; I. crumbly sole horn near the palmar angle; k. medial groove of the frog with thrush.

The sole segment produces again tubular horn, which is quite hard (Figures 1, 7). This tubular horn normally shows a detachment of the horn cells in the distal half of the stratum corneum. But frequently this detachment of horn cells begins more proximal near to the germinative layer, resulting in thin and sensitive soles.

The frog is the anterior part of the heel segment (Figure 7). Both parts produce a relative soft and elastic tubular horn, which allows the lateral extension of the quarters when the hoof is loaded in the stance phase. The frog and heel horn should not become too dry, leading to reduced elasticity and to insufficient hoof mechanism. The frog and heel horn show like the sole horn a normal detachment of horn cells in its distal half. But very frequently a premature decay of these horn cells is seen resulting as thrush (Figures 1, 9).

The growth rate of the hoof horn is different in various parts of the hoof and can be different in breeds and within breeds in individuals, which are housed under the same conditions.

Growth rate	Replacement time
coronary horn, outer zone 7-8 mm/4 weeks	1 year and more
sole horn 5-6 mm/4 weeks	3-4 months

The tensile strength of normal hoof horn varies also under standardized conditions (Küng, 1991).

Tensile strength

coronary horn proximal	– outer zone	60 N/mm^2
	– middle zone	70 N/mm^2
	– inner zone	$40\text{-}55 \text{ N/mm}^2$
coronary horn bearing border		50 N/mm^2 or more
sole horn		55 N/mm^2
frog horn		45 N/mm^2

Feed stuffs and their influence to the hoof horn

Proteins and amino acids

To obtain a good hoof-horn-quality a sufficient protein supply is required. In horses should be sufficient 0.5-1g digestible protein per kg bodyweight for the maintenance, that means 300-400g for a horse of 500-600 kg bodyweight (Meyer, 2002). Supplements of methionine are frequently recommended as well as protein source gelatin or sulfur components as source for the keratin-synthesis.

Carbohydrates

To prevent laminitis carbohydrate-overload should be avoided. Especially the carbohydrates of barley or corn are only incompletely digested in the small intestines. Therefore a great part of soluble carbohydrates can enter into the large intestines, which change the bacterial flora. Fructans may have the same effect. The different types of bacteria may produce toxine, which could damage the capillaries in the soft leaflets or promote a release of a great amount of metalloproteases in this area. Pollitt and collaborators (Pollit and Daradka, 1998; Pass *et al.*, 1998) found that the first changes in the leaflets concern the basement membrane and the stratum basale of the leaflets. Also a diminished glucose supply of these cells may occur (French and Pollitt, 2004). The damage of cells in the soft leaflet area causes the detachment from the soft leaflets to the horn leaflets, and in case of a laminitis the inner part of the hoof sinks down in the horn capsule.

Minerals

The calcium supply will in most regions be sufficiently covered feeding hay and oats. In areas with low calcium content in the soil a supplement should be added (Kempson, 1987). Calcium is needed for the activation of epidermal transglutaminase, which is active in the cross-linkage of the keratin-fibres (Tomlinson *et al.*, 2004).

Zinc is cofactor of more than 200 enzymes, and it is an important factor for maturation of keratinocytes. Measurements of blood plasma content in horses in Switzerland and Austria (mostly fed with hay and oats) frequently indicated that the plasma values were at the lower end of normal plasma values. Coenen and Spitzleik (1996) reported that high doses of 520 mg inorganic zinc per horse and day could improve the hoof condition. In fattening bulls Stern (2000) found that with a supplement of 70 mg organic zinc (Zn-polysacharide, or Zn-proteinate) the hoof condition was significantly improved after 9 months compared to bulls with 70 mg inorganic zinc or unsupplemented controls. Histological investigations of coronary horn revealed that especially in the animals with zinc-proteinate less microcracks could be seen in the coronary horn, which leads to the suggestion that zinc has also an influence on the quality of the intercellular glue, which connects the horn cells. Some observations with a zinc-supplement together with biotin in horses will be presented later.

Copper is cofactor for the activation of thiol-oxidase, which is responsible for the formation of disulfide-bonds in keratins. Up to now, looking at the plasma values, we had no indication of copper deficiency in our horses. Cattle with insufficient copper supply showed more heel cracks, foot rot and sole abscesses (Puls 1984).

Selenium is a coenzyme of the glutathione-peroxidase. The daily need of selenium is near 1.5 mg (500 kg horse, Meyer, 2002). Many nutritional supplements contain selenium. In this case we have to prevent intoxication. After application of too much selenium, decay of the hoof horn near the coronary border was seen (Meyer, 2002). In those cases selenium may be damaging the developing keratinocytes (Tomlinson *et al.*, 2004).

Vitamins

Vitamin A is needed for development and maintenance of epithelial cells and horn tissue. The daily need of about 40'000 units vitamin A (horse of 500 kg bodyweight) will be reached in most diets with a small vitamin supplement.

Biotin

The daily need of biotin is not well known. Meyer (2002) estimates it near 1 mg biotin per horse and day (500 kg bodyweight) or even less. The biotin plasma values of unsupplemented horses are very low. Biotin is coenzyme in many carboxylase enzymes. In Lipizzaner horses with inferior hoof horn quality the tests of carboxylase activities in lymphocytes showed no signs of biotin deficiency (Zenker, 1991). Nevertheless we were able to improve the hoof horn quality in these horses with therapeutic doses of about 20 mg/horse and day (500 kg bodyweight). Experimental induced deficiency was not yet performed in horses. However, experimentally induced biotin deficiency in pigs showed in many cases a dramatic decay of the hoof horn (Geyer *et al.*, 1984). In vitro experiments with a biotin supplement to keratinocytes showed a change in the keratine pattern (Fritsche *et al.*, 1991) compared to unsupplemented cells.

The trials with therapeutic biotin-supplementation in Lipizzaner horses (20 mg per horse and day) showed a good improvement of the hoof horn condition but only with a certain delay to the replacement time of the hoof horn in the different parts of the hooves. The Lipizzaner horses mainly showed cracks in the coronary horn and soft white lines (Figure 9). The hoof horn quality was assessed macroscopically and histologically in bearing border specimens from whom the tensile strength of the coronary horn was tested as well. The macroscopic conditions were improved after 15 months, histology of the bearing border after 19 months and tensile strength of coronary horn from the bearing border beginning from 24 months (Josseck, 1991; Zenker, 1991; Josseck *et al.*, 1995; Zenker *et al.*, 1995).

After 8 years of supplementation the biotin therapy was stopped. After two years the horses reached again a condition, which was poorer than before, which was clearly stated in tensile strength measurements (Munzinger, 2005). Subsequently the horses received a combined supplement containing 20 mg biotine per horse and day, 40 mg zinc-proteinate and 1 g methionine. After 18 months up to 30 months supplementation the horses showed again an improved hoof horn condition. The tensile strength measurements reached significant higher values with the combined supplementation compared to the supplementation with 20 mg biotin alone (Munzinger, 2005).

The diminished number of micro-cracks and minor detachments of horn cells indicate, that biotin, similar as observed with zinc in bulls, may also have a positive influence in the synthesis and quality of the intercellular glue. An improved glue provides better intercellular connections and due to the improved connections less intercellular cracks and higher tensile strength.

Finally it must be stated that the mixture of feces and urine, which surrounds the hooves for a long time, is much more aggressive for hoof horn with damages, like micro-cracks, compared to completely sound horn. Bearing border specimens with micro-cracks which were put for 5 weeks in a mixture of feces and urine showed a dramatic decrease of more than 50% in tensile strength (Munzinger, 2005) compared to sound coronary horn where tensile strength was only slightly and insignificantly diminished after the same treatment with feces and urine (Monhart 2002).

Conclusion

With some nutritional supplements we are able to improve the hoof-horn-condition. But all improvements can only be expected after the renewal time of the hoof horn in the different areas of the hooves.

References

Bolliger, Ch. und H. Geyer (1992), Zur Morphologie und Histochemie des Pferdehufes. Pferdeheilkunde, **8**, 269-286.

Coenen, M. und S. Spitzlei (1996), Zur Zusammensetzung des Hufhorns in Abhängigkeit von Alter, Rasse und Hufhornqualität. Pferdeheilkunde, **12**, 279-283.

French, K.R. and C.C. Pollitt (2004), Equine laminitis: glucose deprivation and MMP activation induce dermo-epidermal separation in vitro. Equine vet. J., **36**, 261-266.

Fritsche, A., G.A. Mathis und F.R. Althaus (1991), Pharmakologische Eirkungen von Biotin auf Epidermiszellen. Schweiz. Arch. Tierheilk., **133**, 277-283.

Geyer, H., J. Schulze, K. Streiff, F. Tagwerker und L. Völker (1984), Der Einfluss des experimentellen Biotinmangels auf Morphologie und Histochemie von Haut und Klaue des Schweines. Zbl. Med. A, **31**, 519-538.

Josseck, H. (1991), Hufhornveränderungen bei Lipizzanerpferden und ein Behandlungsversuch mit Biotin. Diss. med. vet., Zürich.

Josseck, H., W. Zenker und H. Geyer (1995), Hoof horn abnormalities in Lipizzaner horses and the effect of dietary biotin on macroscopic aspects of hoof horn quality. Equine vet. J. **27**, 175-182.

Kempson, S.A. (1987), Scanning electron microscope observations of hoof horn from horses with brittel feet. Vet. Rec. **120**, 568-570.

Küng, M. (1991), Die Zugfestigkeit des Hufhorns von Pferden. Diss. med. vet., Zürich.

Meyer, H. und M. Coenen (2002), Pferdefütterung. 4. Aufl. Parey Buchverlag Berlin

Monhart, B. (2002), Die Einwirkung von Umgebungsfaktoren auf das Hufhorn des Pferdes. Diss. med. vet., Zürich.

Munzinger, K. (2005), Die Hufhornqualität von Lipizzanerpferden und Einflüsse von Futterzusätzen und Umgebungsfaktoren. Diss. med. vet., Zürich.

Pass, M.A., S. Pollitt and C.C. Pollitt (1998), Decreased glucose metabolism causes separation of hoof lamellae in vitro: a trigger for laminitis? Equine vet. J. Suppl. **26**, 133-138.

Pollitt, C.C. and M. Daradka (1998), Equine lamiitis basement membrane pathology: loss of type IV collagen, type VII collagen and laminin immunostaining. Equine vet. J. Suppl. **26**, 139-144.

Puls, R. (1984), Mineral levels in animal health. Diagnostic data. 2nd ed., Sherpa International, Clearbrook, BC, Canada.

Stern, A. (2000), Der Einfluss von Zink auf die Klauenhornqualität von Maststieren. Diss. med. vet., Zürich.

Tomlinson, D.J., C.H. Mülling, and T.M. Fakler (2004), Invited Review: Formation of keratins in the bovine. Claw: Roles of hormones, minerals, and vitamins in functional claw integrity. J. Dairy Sci. **87**, 797-809.

Zenker W. (1991), Hufhornveränderungen bei Lipizzanerpferden und ein Behandlungsversuch mit Biotin. Diss. med. ve.t, Zürich.

Zenker, W., H. Josseck, and H. Geyer (1995), Histological and physical assessment of poor hoof horn quality in Lipizzaner horses and a therapeutic trial with biotin and a placebo. Equine vet. J. **27**, 193-191.

Feeding the endurance horse

Pat Harris

Equine Studies Group, WALTHAM Centre for Pet Nutrition, Melton Mowbray, Leicestershire, United Kingdom

Summary

The endurance horse should be fed for health and vitality during training and the competition rides. OPTIMAL endurance exercise performance is highly dependent on sound nutritional management.
1. Energy provision is key.
   - Feed sufficient energy during training to maintain a body condition score of around 4 (on a 1-9 scale).
   - Forage should be the foundation of all horse diets especially the endurance horse.
   - Avoid very mature hays and it has been suggested that < 30% of the forage should be alfalfa or other high calcium containing hays (although small amounts during training, if maintained during the ride, may be of value). Hay with a low to moderate protein content: 8-14% has been recommended.
   - Alternative higher energy providing fibre sources, 'super fibres' or highly digestible fibre sources, can beneficially be used as part of the diet - e.g. Sugar beet pulp and Soya Hulls.
   - Protein is not a preferred energy source. Excess protein intake may be disadvantageous and it has been recommended that endurance horses should not be fed more than 2g of Digestible Protein/kg Bodyweight/day. Quality and nature of the protein fed however is very important. The lysine and possibly threonine content of the diet of competition/actively exercising horses should be considered.
   - Cereal based feeds will often be needed to maintain energy intake - if using corn use cooked or micronised rather than the unprocessed form. As for all horses small amounts of cereal based feeds should be fed per meal and any changes made gradually.
   - Vegetable oil supplementation has a number of potential performance advantages for the endurance horse and levels of 5-10% in the total diet have been recommended (suggest not more

than 100mls/100kg BW as a guide - add gradually and check the overall mineral, vitamin and protein balance of the resultant diet). Additional Vitamin E at 100-150iu/100mls added oil should be provided above the recommended basal requirement (at 160-250iu/kg DM intake).

2. Adequate water and electrolyte provision is essential.
   - The evaporation of sweat is one of the major mechanisms for the removal of excess heat produced during energy utilisation. Sweat production is accompanied by an obligate loss of electrolytes in particular sodium, potassium and chloride.
   - Horses even with adequate access to water and electrolytes tend to loose 3-7% of their Body Weight during a long ride.
   - Provide adequate sodium and chloride intake during training; sodium, chloride with some calcium and magnesium are advised during a ride
   - No advantage in pre loading with electrolytes days before a race but slight loading on the day of the race may be advantageous.
   - Pastes can be a convenient way to provide electrolytes providing that the horse has adequate access to and drinks water - hypertonic pastes etc. given to dehydrated horses can lead to serious problems.
   - Recently our research has suggested that it may be beneficial not to provide additional potassium supplementation (on top of forage provision) during the ride to certain horses under specific circumstances but it is essential during the recovery period. At present it is therefore recommended, unless specifically advised otherwise, to provide potassium during the ride.

Introduction

Last century saw the horse change from having important roles in the military, agriculture and transportation to becoming part of the expanding leisure industry. A large variety of competitions (show-jumping, endurance, racing, eventing, etc.) have developed to provide a competitive angle to this riding.

At first glance these different competitions have very different demands. Flat racing could be considered to be at one end of the duration/intensity spectrum, with American Quarter horses racing at speeds up to 20 m/s over 400m. In contrast an endurance ride may take place over several days at speeds around 5-6 m/s (on average). Faster speeds during certain stages and rides, however, are now becoming more common especially in some regions e.g. the winner of the 2005 World Equine Endurance Championship race in Dubai covered the 160 km distance at an average speed of around 14 miles per hour ~ 22.5km/hr.

This results in different nutritional demands both in terms of energy and in vitamin and mineral supplementation. However, regardless a horse cannot make it to the Endurance competition or the racetrack without having been healthy and active during its training. This is true for all performance horses regardless of their use and so we should really consider that we are ' *feeding for health and activity'*.

Endurance riding is one of the fastest growing equestrian sports in many developed countries. Endurance horses tend to be lean and muscular; conditioned but not fat; responsive horses without excess energy or excitable behaviour when on the ride and yet with sufficient stamina to complete the ride, at a reasonable speed but without undue stress so that they pass all the Vettings. They also have to be sound and 'tough' both mentally and physically. The effect of any diet on their behaviour is therefore an important consideration and the majority are fed relative to their own temperament, how they are kept, and the nature of the training as well as the type of ride preferred by the rider. This means that, as for other disciplines, there is no single correct way to feed 'an endurance horse' and therefore only general principles can be discussed.

What role can nutrition play?

- Good nutrition will only help a horse to be able to compete optimally; it will not improve the intrinsic ability of the horse (or rider).
- Poor or inappropriate nutrition on the other hand may impose limits on an animal's ability to perform.

Nutrition is particularly important in the endurance horse and endurance riders are in general perhaps the most educated and open-minded group about nutrition of their horses. Why is this?

- There is often plenty of time for nutrition to play a role both in the preparation for the event and during the event itself, which can run over many hours or days.
- Endurance horses are routinely rested and fed during the ride, further increasing the opportunity that nutrition can have to influence performance.
- In an endurance situation nutrients that supply energy can actually be ingested, absorbed, circulated to the muscle and converted to energy whilst the exercise is still being performed.
- The metabolic demands are high requiring the horse to draw heavily on energy reserves and the large sweat fluid losses mean that aggressive replacement strategies are required to keep the horse hydrated.
- The majority of clinical problems especially in the upper level of competition horses, other than lameness *per se*, tend to be metabolic conditions such as tying up, loss of appetite due to stress and long term training, dehydration during heavy training with sweat and fluid loss and poor recovery after hard competition. Depletion of energy reserves, dehydration and electrolyte imbalances can all contribute to poor performance and fatigue. In an overview of ~7000 starts on international races only 50% completed the ride with 30% being eliminated - 63% because of lameness, 24% for metabolic reasons and 13% for other causes. Appropriate nutritional management may help reduce the incidence of elimination especially for metabolic reasons.

Optimal endurance exercise performance, therefore, is highly dependent on sound nutritional management.

Why is energy supply and utilisation so important?

The supply of energy is crucial for life and movement. In general terms if a horse is fed too little energy for its needs it will tend to become dull and lethargic and/or lose weight and/or become clinically ill. If a horse is fed too much energy or inappropriate energy it may become hyperactive and/or gain weight and/or become ill.

Endurance horses are commonly asked to undertake low intensity, long duration exercise and the ability to do this is highly dependent on body stores of fuel in the form of both glycogen and fat. As diet can affect the type and amount of fuel that horses can store as well as their ability to use such fuels effectively and efficiently, manipulating the diet can therefore influence how soon fatigue develops and whether the animal can complete the ride or not. Endurance ride body condition was assessed in one study and the average BCS on a 1-9 scale was 4.67 and the % of body fat, predicted from rump fat thickness using ultrasound, was 7.8%. The top finishers had an estimated 6.5% body fat and the non-finishers 11% body fat. In another one looking at the 100mile Tevis cup (Garlinghouse and Burrill, 1999) the BCS of horses pre ride was 4.5 (on a 1-9 scale) for those which completed the ride and no horse with a BCS of < 3 completed. Horses, which were eliminated for non-metabolic reasons such as lameness and going over the time, had a pre ride mean BCS of ~4.5 compared to a mean BCS of ~2.9 for horses which were eliminated for metabolic failure. These results may not be applicable to all endurance events but they suggest that at least in the more difficult rides thin horses with a CS of less than 3 might be at a disadvantage because of lower energy reserves. In addition, it was suggested that over-conditioned horses could have problems due to the insulating effect etc. of a thicker fat cover.

Energy is supplied to the horse via its diet but fundamentally energy is not a nutrient. The chemical energy or gross energy contained within feeds needs to be converted into a form of energy that the cells can use for mechanical work or movement (useable or net energy). Ultimately the 'currency' used to fuel this movement is Adenosine Triphosphate (ATP). In order to exercise for a prolonged period of time effectively, ideally for the majority of the ride ATP must be re-synthesised at a similar rate at which it is being used. Stored energy, in the form of muscle and liver glycogen, intramuscular and adipose triglycerides, along with energy derived from the feed ingested during longer rides are used to provide this ATP production. At certain speeds, under steady state conditions, the ATP used can be regenerated by oxidative phosphorylation or aerobic metabolism of fats and glucose. Aerobic metabolism of fats is very efficient as far as ATP production is concerned but it is comparatively slow compared to the breakdown of glycogen especially by anaerobic means - therefore as the speed of exercise increases anaerobic breakdown of Glycogen becomes increasing important. This enables exercise to continue but results in lactic acid accumulation, which contributes to fatigue. Typical speeds for endurance used to be within the range that can be maintained almost entirely through aerobic energy production - only during controlled runaways that some riders use at the beginning or at the end 'race 'sprint' or when hill climbing does energy production shift towards anaerobic means and then ideally only for a short period of time. However, this is changing as speeds during certain loops and rides increase.

Fat stores are comparatively large and therefore fatigue in an endurance horse is primarily caused, it is currently believed, by depletion of the glycogen stores (combined with fluid and electrolyte disturbances). However, much more research is needed in this whole area.

Energy requirements

The actual energy requirements for an endurance horse will depend on the speed that it is being ridden as well as the terrain etc. but in general terms it will reflect:

- Maintenance requirements plus an allowance for the work
- Maintenance using the NRC (Martin Rosset *et al.*, 1994) = 4.184 x (1.4 + 0.03xBody weight) MJ/day. Which for a 450Kg endurance horse would be around 62 MJ

The amount for the ride - training or competition - would depend on the weight of the horse plus rider and tack as well as the speed of work as illustrated in Table 1 (adapted from 3). So if the horse with an extra 75Kg for the rider and tack was given a training ride for 3hrs at a medium trot then it would have an estimated additional energy requirement of around 62MJ giving a total requirement of 124MJ for that day. This fits very well with a survey of the feeding practices of a group of riders participating in training clinics for aspiring international competitors in the US (Crandell, 2002) where average estimated daily intakes during training were around 100MJ. Obviously higher intakes would be needed during the competition - although it should be appreciated that not all the energy expended will be replenished during the competition. In addition, horses are individuals and therefore even those undertaking the same amount and type of work may each require not only a different amount of energy but also a different way of supplying it. The aim being to feed the horse during training to maintain a body CS of around 4.

Table 1. A guide to potential Digestible Energy (DE) requirements above Maintenance at various speeds.

Gait	Speed (meters/min)	DE MJ/Kg BW (of horse plus rider plus tack)/hr
Slow walk	59	0.0071
Fast Walk	95	0.0105
Slow Trot	200	0.0272
Medium Trot	250	0.03975
Fast Trot/slow canter	300	0.0573
Medium Canter	350	0.0816

How best to provide this energy

Dietary energy is provided to the horse by four principal dietary energy sources (see also Figure 1):

1. Hydrolysable carbohydrates, e.g. simple sugars & starch. These can be digested by mammalian enzymes to hexoses which are absorbed from the small intestine (SI) or if they 'escape' digestion in the SI they are rapidly fermented in the hindgut. This can lead to clinical problems such as laminitis and colic.
2. Fermentable fibres, component of dietary fibre e.g., Cellulose, pectins, hemicelluloses etc. These are not digestible by mammalian enzymes but can be fermented by the microorganisms predominantly located in the hindgut. Speed of fermentation as well as site may play an important role in the energy value to the horse.
3. Oils/Fats, Despite their more 'evolutionary traditional' diet containing relatively low concentrations of oils, horses in general appear to be able to digest and utilise up to 20% of their diet as oil if suitably introduced.
4. Proteins. Not a nutritionally preferred option as an energy source: it is inefficiently converted to useable energy with proportionally higher amounts of waste energy (heat) produced; the nitrogen must be removed, as excess protein is not stored, resulting in increased water requirements as the excess protein is lost primarily as urea in the urine; and potentially higher ammonia levels in the stable as the urea is converted by bacteria in the environment to ammonia.

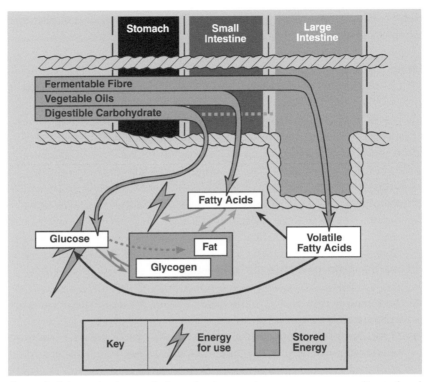

Figure 1. Schematic picture of where the three main energy sources are digested and how the end products of digestion are utilized. © WALTHAM

Different feeds and feedstuffs contain differing amount of the raw chemical energy and the efficiency of their conversion to useable or net energy also differs widely (Harris, 1997). Cereals have more net energy than hay does; hay contains more than twice the net or useable energy than straw. Hay produces much more spare 'lost' heat than do cereals so is much more 'internally heating'. Vegetable oils contain proportionally more net energy than the cereals (~2.5 times as much digestible energy as maize/corn and 3 times as much as oats).

Forage is the foundation

Forage should be the foundation of all horse diets especially the endurance horse. In a recent survey of top riders in the US (Crandell,

2002) at least 80% of the horses had 24-hr turnout (with additional preserved forage at times of the year). The average forage content of the diets was 78%, which is much higher in comparison to other types of sports horses (e.g. Racehorses may be 30% or even less).

- The horse evolved to live on forage based diets and is best suited to such a diet.
- Volatile Fatty Acids: the endpoint of fibre fermentation are absorbed from the hindgut and transported to the liver where they can be converted to glucose and stored as liver glycogen (important in maintaining blood glucose levels during exercise) or converted to fat used to support the body's fat stores. During an endurance race the horse must use other sources for the formation of glucose in order to save the glycogen stores which can only be replenished slowly. Fibre can be used as an energy source throughout the endurance ride since fermentation of fibre and absorption of VFAs continues long after the fibre has been eaten. Proprionic acid from the hindgut fermentation of fibre is probably the most important precursor for glucose (although glycerol from the breakdown of body fat may also be important).
- A forage-based diet provides the horse with a fluid and electrolyte reservoir in the gut which it can draw on during exercise. Work has shown that a diet high in fibre results in an increased water intake - plus horses supplemented with a simple hay and salt diet had 73% more water in their digestive tracts after exercise and approximately 33% more available electrolytes than those on a low fibre diet. This is believed to be due to the high water holding capacity of plant fibre.
- High fibre/forage diets help maintain gut health (incl. reducing risk gastric ulcers and maintaining hind gut health) as well as psychological well being. The presence of fibre in the digestive system has been said to help maintain a good blood flow to the various tissues and perhaps help prevent colic.

Current recommended practical hints

- Avoid feeding very mature forages.
- Select hay with a low to moderate protein content - 8-14% has been recommended.
- It is often recommended to avoid high intakes of high calcium containing forages (and if provided during training should consider

providing during the ride) e.g. suggested by some that less than 50% of the forage should be alfalfa and preferably less than 30%.
■ A good quality grass hay can be ideal or a grass hay (predominant) /alfalfa mix.

Cereal addition

Forage, as explained above, is unlikely to be able to provide sufficient energy for prolonged exercise. Many endurance horses are Arabian, at least in part, and tend to be 'easy' keepers. However, even quality pasture/preserved forage will often not enable endurance horses to maintain weight when they begin heavy work. Therefore, some cereals are often added into most endurance horse diets especially when in hard training - the average amount in the endurance survey (Coenen, 2002) was 2.27kg /day.

Popping, flaking, or micronising of corn/maize can be very advantageous to maximise the useable energy obtained from the feed. The use of processed corn can be advantageous especially in the smaller framed horses where you wish to reduce the bulk of the feed being fed but maximise the energy provided by the cereals. The relationship between weight and volume, as shown below, varies between the cereals, e.g. oats weigh less for a given volume than corn so if measured in volumes you, will effectively, be feeding less weight of oats and far less actual energy.

As for all horses it is preferable to feed small amounts of cereal based feeds (e.g. < 0.4kg/100kg BW/meal in a grain-adapted horse) as often

Table 2. A comparison of cereals and their energy content by volume and weight.

Feed	Kg/L i.e. Vol.	Digestible Energy - MJ/kg	Relative feeding value to corn by weight	Relative feeding value to corn by volume
Corn	0.8	14.2	100	100
Oats - regular	0.4	11.7	85	45
Oats- naked	0.7	15.9	110	95
Barley	0.7	13.8	95	85

as is required to provide the necessary energy intake - consider alternative energy sources such as alternative fibres and/or vegetable oil.

Alternative fibre based energy sources

As described above cereals provide more net energy than does forage. However, the upper part of the gastrointestinal tract has a relatively small capacity and the horse has digestive and metabolic limitations to high grain, starch and sugar based diets. Large grain meals may overwhelm the digestive capacity of the stomach and small intestine leading to the rapid fermentation of the grain carbohydrate in the hindgut. This potentially can result in one of a number of disorders including colic, diarrhoea and laminitis. High starch based diets are also not suitable for most horses that are prone to Tying-up etc. (Harris and Kronfeld, 2003). Therefore, there has been increasing interest in the use of alternative energy sources for horses especially alternative fibre sources, which do not cause such marked disturbances in the hindgut and yet provide more energy than typical forages. These tend to have a high content of fibre that can be fermented and low levels of relatively indigestible material such as lignin. Examples of these include sugar beet pulp and Soya hulls. Sugar beet pulp may also assist with water status due to its potential ability to hold large amounts of water in the GIT tract and therefore act as a good reservoir.

Oil supplementation can be very beneficial

Our relatively recent research (Pagan *et al.*, 1997) has shown that in Arabians undertaking low intensity exercise feeding an oil supplemented diet ($\sim 29\%$ of the DE from oil) was associated with beneficial alterations in the metabolic response to the exercise including:

- More than 30% reduction in the production and utilization of glucose after 5 and 10 weeks of feeding the oil supplemented diet.
- A decrease in the Respiratory Exchange ratio after 5-10 weeks.
- A decrease in the estimated rate of whole body carbohydrate utilization attributable to decreases in muscle glycogen and plasma glucose utilization.
- An increase in the whole body rate of lipid oxidation during exercise - beneficial during prolonged exercise.

Vegetable oil supplemented diets have the following potential advantages:

■ The increase in the energy density of the feed effectively means more fibre can often be fed and less cereals or hydrolysable starch - whilst still maintaining the desired energy intake. This in turn helps to maintain the microfloral population in the hindgut and prevent over production, in particular, of lactic acid, which could lead to digestive and other metabolic disturbances (Harris and Kronfeld, 2003).

■ Long term (~5weeks plus) oil supplementation in combination with appropriate training, however, has been proposed to result in the following adaptations which could result in improved performance (see also 6,17):

  □ Increased mobilisation of free fatty acids (FFA) and increased speed of mobilisation.

  □ Increased speed of uptake of FFA into muscle (Orme *et al.*, 1997) - often considered to be rate limiting.

  □ A glycogen sparing effect so that fatigue is delayed and performance improved - could be especially important in endurance activities.

  □ Increased pre-exercise muscle glycogen levels.

■ Some researchers have suggested that horses fed an oil supplemented diet retain a higher percentage of absorbed water than when fed a hay only diet and that packed cell volumes during exercise are lower even though sweating losses are higher, suggesting a greater reserve of water in the extracellular fluid (Matjoaspn-Kochan *et al.*, 1994).

■ Less bowel ballast which can then be balanced by the increase in fibre (which creates more bowel ballast) resulting in no effective change although the horse effectively has more water holding capacity than a non-oil/higher starch fed horse.

■ In a similar way as oil in the diet is more efficiently converted to useable energy than feeds such as hay and cereals this may reduce the heat load on the horse, which may be particularly useful when competing under hot and humid conditions - this reduction helps balance any increase in fibre (which increases the heat load).

■ Less bulk has to be fed to maintain intake which can be important in some endurance horses which may have either a reduced capacity for bulky feeds or have limits on appetite imposed by the stress of extended exercise in preparation for competition.

- Behavioural advantages - horses fed oil supplemented diets rather than high starch based diets tend to be calmer (Holland *et al.*, 1996).
- Feeding a low starch, high fibre diet, (which is supplemented if necessary with oil) is recommended for the feeding of horses that are prone to suffering from Tying up which is a not uncommon problem in Endurance horses.

Practical hints

- Supplemental fat or oil diets can be supplied in four main ways:
  1. As a vegetable oil supplemented manufactured diet - the advantage here is that such diets should come ready balanced with respect to the protein, vitamins and minerals intake that they provide when fed with forage (and as required salt). Can be a simple, practical and convenient way to feed high fat diets. *Adding oil to the diet has the potential for creating multiple imbalances and therefore where possible the use of appropriately supplemented or fortified diets are preferred.*
  2. High fat supplemental feedstuffs - (such as rice bran), which are also high in fibre and usually low in starch. However, some of the rice brans available have the same disadvantages of wheat bran in that they have a very imbalanced Calcium to Phosphorus content.
  3. Supplemental animal fat - many horses find most animal fats to be unpalatable and they seem often to be more likely to cause digestive upsets. Their use is not to be recommended.
  4. Supplemental vegetable oils - such as corn oil or Soya oil. Different ways of processing may affect palatability.
- Any supplemental oil or oil supplemented feed should be introduced slowly and should be fresh and not rancid. Dietary fats are usually hydrolysed in the small intestine and the capacity to hydrolyse lipids seems to adapt in herbivores over a week or two. Horses have been shown to be able to digest and utilise up to 20% of the diet as oil although around 10% of the daily intake has been suggested by some in the literature to provide the maximal beneficial metabolic effects. Levels of ~ 5 % in the total diet are more common in some high performing/endurance horses and many horses (~ 450kg BW) can be fed up to 400mls (~ 370g) daily in divided doses without any problems - provided that it has been introduced gradually and is not

rancid. It is important to balance the overall diet to ensure an adequate intake of vitamins, minerals and protein.

Interestingly despite work to suggest that around 5- 10% of the diet as oil may be the most beneficial for endurance, only just over half of the horses in the endurance (Crandell, 2002) survey were receiving additional oil in the form of oil or rice bran. The average oil percentage in this survey was only 2.3% and ranged from as low as 1.45 to as high as 6.9%.

- It is very important to note that supplemental oil does not provide any additional protein, vitamins (Vitamin E level variable) or minerals. If the horse is not receiving sufficient, for its work load, from its basal diet, then an appropriate additional mix may be needed (usually it is helpful to contact the Nutritional Helpline of the feed being fed and inform them of the diet and workload, and get direct advice appropriate for their supplement) or consider a manufactured, balanced, high oil feed.
- It is recommended that additional Vitamin E be fed in combination with any supplemental Vegetable oil. Exact recommendations are not known but an additional (above requirements see below) 100iu Vitamin E/100mls of added supplemental oil is the author's current recommendation.

When should you exercise in relation to a meal?

There has been considerable debate across the years about when and what should be fed horses before they are exercised and/or at a competition. Should they be fed or fasted and when should the hay be fed in relation to the grain and/or exercise? Several studies have shown that a pre-exercise concentrate meal suppresses free fatty acid (FFA) availability and increases blood glucose disappearance during exercise but these did not necessarily look at the influence of forage on these responses. It is even more complex for an endurance horse because not only are they fed during longer rides where there is a great influence of exercise induced hormones which may counterbalance the effect of hormones induced by any feeding occasion.

In conclusion at this moment in time the recommendation appears to be: Try not to start to exercise close to feeding a large concentrate/grain rich meal, which is based on the following:

- Glucose peaks around 1-3 hrs past a meal, which is associated with a rise in Insulin. Insulin promotes glycogen formation in the liver, fat storage and protein synthesis in the muscles - in particular it suppresses fat oxidation - i.e. promotes storage not use of energy. Exercising at this point may result in a drop in blood glucose during the first stages of exercise which may not be desirable (the brain can only use glucose as a fuel) and may retard the release of free fatty acids into the circulation (so the horse has to rely even more on stored glycogen - potentially resulting in a quicker onset of fatigue). This becomes less of an issue once the ride has begun because the effects of insulin may be countered to a certain extent by adrenaline and cortisol (induced by exercise) and thyroxine.
- A large amount of fluid, which comes effectively from the circulating blood, is secreted into the gut during digestion. With large concentrate meals, especially in quick or greedy feeders, there can be up to 24% loss in plasma volume within the first hour following feeding. Exercising under these conditions would effectively be like working a dehydrated horse.

Much more work is needed before detailed guidance can be given for the optimal recommendations for the endurance horse before or during a ride.

What about protein requirements?

Additional protein over maintenance may be needed with exercise and training because of the accompanying muscular development, the need for muscle repair and to replenish the nitrogen lost in sweat. The precise protein requirements for exercise, however, are unknown and the current NRC recommendations are 9, 10.4 and 11% crude protein in the total ration for horses in light, moderate and intense exercise respectively (NRC, 1989). In the endurance (Crandell, 2002) survey the overall protein content of the diets averaged 10.2% but ranged from 6.2-15.7% depending mainly on the type of forage offered. Excessive protein is particularly undesirable for the endurance horse as outlined above and it has been recommended that endurance horses should not be fed more than 2g of Digestible Protein/kg Bodyweight/day

Quality and nature of the protein fed is important especially in growing horses and those in hard or repetitive work. The lysine and possibly threonine content of the diet of competition/actively exercising horses should be considered - Soya bean meal/flakes are, for example, a good source of lysine. The amount of additional lysine needed will depend on the hay and pasture being fed as for example alfalfa and other legumes are higher in lysine than many meadow hays and grasses. NRC currently recommends lysine in g/day at 0.035 x Crude Protein requirements (g/day) for horses in work whose crude protein requirements are given as ~10g/MJ energy/day.

Can diet help my horse run longer and faster?

An ergogenic aid can be considered to be any factor which can increase or improve work production. This could result in an increase in speed, or endurance or strength and therefore could potentially improve performance of the endurance horse. Possible ways that ergogenic aids, apart from equipment etc., could improve performance in the horse could include (see also 7):

- Psychological effects.
- Improved co-ordination or recruitment of muscle fibres.
- Provision of a supplementary fuel source or the feeding of a feed with a higher energy content.
- Increased levels of available stored energy.
- Improved efficiency of conversion of the chemical energy of the feed, or stored energy, to mechanical energy for work.
- Improved ATP/ADP homeostasis in contracting muscle fibres.
- Decreased substrate depletion.
- Decreased end product accumulation including improved intra-cellular acid base regulation.

These could result in increased mechanical energy for work and/or a delayed onset of fatigue or improved neuromuscular co-ordination. Vegetable oil supplementation could be considered a natural ergogenic aid in the endurance horse. Many other substances have theoretical ergogenic properties and there is insufficient space to discuss more than one of these here. Certainly the carbohydrate based nutritional strategies employed by human marathon runners do not appear to be of any value for the equine endurance horse. Dietary supplied Branch Chain Amino Acids (alanine, valine, leucine and isoleucine) have been suggested to be able to affect performance by increasing the rate of energy production via the TCA cycle, as well as having an effect on factors contributing to central fatigue. Whilst BCCA supplements are available to the human athlete, data on their ergogenic effect following oral ingestion is contradictory. In a human study, a positive effect on metabolism (increased alanine synthesis, reduced fall in muscle glutamate, and lower glycogen utilisation during exercise) was apparent and were favourable to an increase in endurance performance. However other studies have not been so positive. Recent work in the horse, for example, has failed to show any effect of BCAA supplementation in conditioned animals (see 19) on performance although these did not evaluate the role specifically in endurance races. Certainly changes in plasma concentrations have been recorded for horses during a simulated 60km race (Trottier *et al.*, 1997). It is also possible that they may have more of a role to play during recovery rather than during the competition itself. Further work is obviously needed in this area before any recommendations can be given.

What about salt and other electrolytes?

Unfortunately the conversion of chemical energy provided by the feed to mechanical energy in the form of ATP that can be used by the muscles is not very efficient and the 'waste' heat that is produced has to be removed from the body. One of the main mechanisms for heat remove is via the evaporation of sweat (Coenen, 2002) . The amount of sweat produced depends on the environmental conditions, nature of the work (which in turn will depend on the rider's ability and the terrain) and the animal's fitness. Under favourable climate conditions, sweat loss can be around 2-5L/hr if run at a low pace (~ 2-4m/s) or in the order of 7-8 L/hr in long distance rides ridden at a faster pace/difficult terrain. In hot humid conditions where sweating is partially ineffective production can be as high as 10-15L/hr. Sweat production seems to only decrease after extreme water loss and although there may be some changes in sweat composition with time basically sweat production is accompanied by an obligate loss of electrolytes. When the sweat loss is low much of the loss can be made up by absorption of water contained in the large intestine but if water losses are greater (3-4% BW) a decrease in circulatory volume as well as a loss of skin elasticity occurs. Horses participating in endurance rides over distances of 50 - 200km typically lose 3-7% of their body weight during the competition - some horses may lose up to 10%. These loses are only partially compensated for during overnight stops - perhaps due to persistent loss in the GIT content which takes longer than an overnight period to recover to pre race levels (Schott *et al.*, 1997).

Sweat contains relatively low levels of calcium ($\sim$0.12g/L), magnesium ($\sim$ 0.05g/l) and phosphate (<0.01g/L) bur relatively high levels of sodium, potassium and chloride as shown in Table 3. There are also small amounts of various trace elements e.g. Iron at $\sim$4.3mg/L and Zn at 11.4mg/L. However, the main electrolytes lost with sweat are sodium, potassium and chloride.

Table 3. A guide to the sodium, potassium and chloride content of equine sweat.

Electrolyte	Approx. concentration in one litre of Sweat g/L	Approximate amount that would need to be ingested to replace the amount lost in one litre of sweat - g
Sodium (Na)	3.1	3.45
Potassium (K)	1.6	2
Chloride (Cl)	5.3	5.5

Electrolytes are critical nutrients for all horses but particularly the endurance horse - as they play an important role in maintaining osmotic pressure, fluid balance and muscle activity. Fluid accompanied by electrolyte losses can therefore result in major clinical problems. The exhausted horse syndrome, not uncommon in endurance events, is an extreme example and is believed to reflect a combination of fluid and electrolyte losses, depletion of energy stores and extremes of environmental conditions.

Supplementation during training

In an endurance horse the forage-based diet should provide an adequate reserve for potassium and therefore the main concern should be for salt replenishment. The sodium requirements for a horse at rest have been estimated at 20mg/kg/day (assuming that the sodium sources are 90% available). It has been suggested that the sodium requirements for exercise should take into consideration the sodium content of sweat and the amount needed to be fed to replace this ($\sim$3.45 g/L for replacement) and the amount of sweat produced i.e. suggested for light, moderate, hard and very heavy exercise around 0.5 -1, 1-2, 2-5 & 7-8 L/100kg bodyweight or the rates given above per hour of work.

As an example: a 450 kg endurance horse which is in training work, and does 3hrs of training work (counted as low end of hard work above -i.e. 2L/100kg BW or sweating at a rate of 3L/hr), in temperate conditions may be estimated as losing 9 l of sweat.

Estimated requirements would be:

Maintenance (20mg/kgBW)	= 9g
+ For the Sweat (replacement)	= 9 x 3.45g $\sim$ 31
Total $\sim$40g of Sodium (equivalent to around 3.5oz of salt).	

It should however be noted that this method of determining sodium requirements most likely overestimates daily requirements of horses, especially those that are sweating considerably, as the content of the gastrointestinal tract provides an important reservoir for sodium during hard work and therefore the electrolyte losses that occur with sweating may not need to be restored all at once. It is therefore worthwhile considering the weekly loss of electrolytes and then determining an average amount of sodium that should be provided on a daily basis. However, all the above recommendations are only guidelines, which have to be adjusted to the individual horse and situation; often professional advice should be acquired.

Most complementary feeds, and home mixed rations, do not provide sufficient sodium and chloride intake for horses that are significantly losing these electrolytes in sweat. Salt should be provided, therefore, to many horses in work. Horses may eat up to the amount stated above when provided with free choice salt or in some cases a salt block. However, intake particularly with a block cannot be guaranteed. In general, in the 2002 endurance survey (Crandell, 2002) only 35% of the riders overall offered horses free choice access to salt but there were extreme differences between regions with 75% of the East coast riders offering salt but only 16% of the West coast. Only 5% fed a daily electrolyte - although they all fed electrolytes during a ride.

For those horses in little or no work the provision of a salt block may be adequate (but ensure that it is sited so that its use by that individual horse can be monitored). Where complementary feed or a vitamin mineral supplement is being fed, any block should be a pure salt rather than a mineralised one. It is not advised that owners use blocks formulated for other species. For those horses in more work or who sweat noticeably the recommendation is that additional salt should be added to the feed - unless you have monitored and confirmed that your individual horse is eating sufficient from a block etc. Salt should only be introduced or removed from a feed gradually. By providing the supplementary sodium as salt you are likely to maintain chloride intake at a reasonable level.

It is important to note that in various references within the literature, slightly different amounts of sodium may be recommended for the various workloads. This may in part occur because each of these references allow for slightly different amounts of sodium in sweat, estimate different amounts of sweat that each level workload will produce as well vary in the level of availability of sodium that they use.

Practical hint

A very rough estimate of the amount of sweat an individual horse has lost can be made by accurately weighing the horse before and after exercise (and before the horse drinks). Approximately 0.9L of fluid has been lost for every 1kg loss in bodyweight. (NB have to allow for any faecal or urinary losses).

Feeding strategies around race days

Pre ride

■ Training tends to be light in the 4-5 days before a race - which combined with regular feeding will help to ensure that the glycogen stores are 'topped' up.
■ As discussed above you want to have a gut filled with water and forage - so forage intake should be high before a ride and use good quality forage during the ride.
■ Allow the horse to nibble on hay or other forage in the hours before the race starts.

- It has been suggested that a high glycaemic meal the night before may be helpful to top up liver glycogen stores - but do not overload the small intestine (< 2kg sweet feed/meal for 500kg horse which has been adapted to having grain feeds).
- No information to support the use of electrolyte loading over the days pre a race as they are likely to be quickly excreted within a few hours.
- Calcium and magnesium may compete for uptake etc so ensure that the calcium intake is not too high and that there is sufficient magnesium being provided.

Day of the race

- Electrolytes given a few hours before a prolonged exercise competition may be of value if adequate water is also provided and the horses are adequately hydrated - do not give excessive amounts of electrolytes.
- Glycerol administration does not seem to be of value and may in fact increase water electrolyte loss.
- Pastes can be a convenient way to provide electrolytes providing that the horse has adequate access to and drinks water - such hypertonic pastes given to dehydrated horses can lead to serious problems.
- Recently our research has suggested that it may be beneficial not to provide additional potassium supplementation (on top of forage provision) during the ride *to certain horses under specific circumstances* but it is essential during the recovery period. At present it is therefore recommended unless specifically advised otherwise to provide potassium during the ride (Hess *et al.*, 2003).
- Small amounts of Calcium, and magnesium supplementation during the ride are recommended but predominantly sodium and chloride.
- If the aim is to maximise digestion in the hind gut during exercise it has been suggested that pellets or cubes would be type of feed to feed because they are consumed faster, have a faster stomach and intestine passage time - but there has been some resistance to pelleted feed.
- There are in fact no hard and fast rules on what to feed during a race - it does depend to a large extent on what the horse will eat - certainly it should be offered high quality feedstuffs and plenty of water. Mash or slurry mixtures are popular including materials such as alfalfa

meal, cereals, wheat bran/rice bran plus some molasses with succulents to encourage eating. Most also provide plain forage (often soaked). Some recommend adding some electrolytes to the feed if this does not discourage eating or waiting until the horse has eaten and drunk to give any electrolyte pastes.

Post ride

- Water immediately.
- Free choice hay followed by some cereal or mash (as per the ride) then maintain on normal diet for the next few days - do not attempt to replenish all the lost energy in the immediate post ride period.
- Provide supplementary electrolytes over the 24hr post race period - include Potassium in this supplement.

Water should be provided *ad lib* and horses trained to take any opportunity to drink. Water should be offered at frequent intervals during a ride - e.g. every 30-40 mins especially in hot weather.

What about vitamin E, selenium and other antioxidants?

Free radical reactions are responsible for many key biochemical events and under controlled circumstances they are essential for life but when uncontrolled they can cause the irreversible denaturation of essential cellular components and can result in a number of degenerative disease processes. Free radical induced damage has been associated with processes including ageing, as well as joint, muscle and respiratory disease. A system of natural antioxidant defences is present in the body to help counteract such free radical induced damage, including the selenium containing enzyme, glutathione peroxidase and Vitamin E. GSHPx for example acts to reduce the production of hydroxyl radicals. Vitamin E acts as a scavenger of free radicals and Vitamin C may assist by reducing the tocpheroxyl radicals formed by this scavenging. In addition, Vitamin E helps to block lipid peroxidation and may also form an important part of membrane structure. During exercise there is a marked increase in free radical production in the horse due in particular to the increased activity of xanthine oxidase during anaerobic degradation of purine nucleotides and the partial reduction of oxygen during oxidative phosphorylation within the mitochondria. It is thought that free radical production may play a role in muscle damage and fatigue of exercise if the production exceeds the capacity of the cells' natural defence mechanisms. All horses, but especially those in hard work such as the endurance horse need Vitamin E and selenium.

Our research has shown that the levels of antioxidants throughout an endurance race depend to some extent on the difficulty of the race and the environmental conditions. The work suggests that antioxidant supplementation before and during the race may be beneficial (5,11). Despite all of this only 19% in the 2002 endurance survey (Crandell, 2002) fed a vitamin and Se supplement (none on the West and Central regions but 67% on the East Coast. This may reflect the fact that the soils and forages are very deficient in the East Coast).

The NRC (NRC, 1989) recommends as a minimum for horses in work: - Vitamin E: 80iu/kg DM intake/day. The author's recommendation is at least double this figure at 160iu/kg DM intake plus additional Vitamin E to support any supplemental oil (see above). For Selenium the NRC recommends as a minimum for horses in work: 0.1mg/kg DM intake/day. The author's recommendation again is twice this at 0.2mg/kg DM intake and not to exceed in the total ration more than 1mg Selenium /100kg BW/day.

Conclusions

Appropriate nutrition during the training period and the race itself can help to minimise certain metabolic problems. It is therefore very important for all those involved in this complex sport to have a good understanding of nutritional practices.

References

Coenen M., 2002. Exercise and stress - Impact on adaptive processes involving water and electrolytes In Nutrition of the performance horse an international perspective. Proc of the 2002 KER equine Nutrition Conference. 113-134

Crandell K., 2002. Trends in feeding the American Endurance horse in Proc of the 2002 KER Equine nutrition conference 135-139

Garlinghouse S.E. and Burrill M.J., 1999. Relationship of body condition score to completion rate during 160km endurance races Equine Veterinary Journal suppl 30 591-595.

Harris P.A., 1997 Energy sources and requirements of the exercising horse *Annu. Rev. Nutr.* 17, 185 - 210.

Harris P.A. and Kronfeld, 2003. Influence of dietary energy sources on Health and performance. Current therapy in equine medicine 5 Robinson NE (ed) Saunders Philadelphia 698 -704.

Hess T.M., K. Greiwe-Crandell J.E., Waldron, D.S. Kronfeld and Harris, P.A., 2003. Potassium-free electrolytes and calcium supplementation in an endurance race. *Proc . 18th Equine Nutrition and Physiology symposium 146-147*

Holland *et al.*, 1996 Behavior of horses is affected by soy lecithin and corn oil in the diet. *J Anim Sci* 74 1252 - 1255.

Martin Rosset W, Vermorel M, Doreau M, Tisserand JL, Andrieu, 1994. The French horse feed evaluation systems and recommended allowances for energy and protein. *Livestock Production Sci.* 40: 37-56.

Matjoaspn-Kochan K.J., Potter G.D., Caggiano S. and Michael E.M., 2001. Ration digestibility , water balance and physiologic responses in horses fed varying diets and exercised in hot weather ENPS 261-266.

NRC, 1989. *Nutrient requirements of horses* 5th edition. Washington DC. National Academy press .

Orme C.E., Harris R.C., Marlin D.J. and Hurley J.S., 1997. Metabolic adaptation to a fat supplemented diet in the thoroughbred horse *Br J Nutr.*,**78**, 443-458.

Pagan J.D., Geor R.J., Harris P.A., Hoekstra K., Grdner S., Hudson C. and Prine A., 2002. Effects of fat adaptation on glucose kinetics and substrate oxidation during low intensity exercise. Equine Vet J Suppl. 34 33-38.

Schott H.C., McGlade K.S., Hines M.T. and Petersen A., 1997. Body weight , fluid and electrolyte, and hormonal changes in horses that successfully completed a five day, 424 kilometre endurance competition. Equine Athlete 40 -44.

Trottier N.L., Nielsen, Lang K.L., Ku. and Schott, 2002. Equine Endurance exercise alters serum branched chain amino acid and alanine concentrations. Equine Vet J 34 168-172

Impact of nutrition on the microflora of the gastro-intestinal tract in horses

Véronique Julliand
ENESAD, 21079 Dijon, France, v.julliand@enesad.fr

Introduction

Various microorganisms in high levels inhabit the gastro-intestinal tract (GIT) of horses and interact with each other in a series of complex relations. These microorganisms are essential inhabitants of the different compartments of the normal and healthy GIT and influence nutritional processes as well as the digestive health of the host. The breakdown of plant cell-walls has been investigated in the hindgut and appears very similar to that described in ruminants. Conversely nutrition of their host has a major impact on the GI microorganisms and contributes to control their balance within the GI ecosystem. As a matter of fact feeding the horse in the respect of its GI microbes appears as a real challenge. Choosing the ration of horses is all the more difficult for athletic horses because they receive highly energetic diets, fed in two or three meals rather than spread all day. This has an impact on the GI microbial ecology and consequently can even lead to disorders.

The response to dietary treatment has been studied experimentally and appeared to be highly variable: favorable for optimizing the utilization of plant cell-wall in some cases (Julliand *et al.*, 2001), the diet can become drastic under extreme feeding practices, leading to colic or laminitis (Garner *et al.*, 1978). Interestingly, epidemiological studies have confirmed that nutrition may be a factor predisposing to colic in horses. Feeding hay in round bales was reported as a risk factor for colic (Hudson *et al.*, 2001). Supplying relatively large amounts of concentrate also appeared to increase the risk for developing colic (Hudson *et al.*, 2001; Reeves *et al.*, 1996; Tinker *et al.*, 1997). The feeding treatment affecting the most the risk of colic was changes: changes in type of concentrate, type or batch of hay, or pasture grass (Hudson *et al.*, 2001; Reeves *et al.*, 1996; Tinker *et al.*, 1997; Proudman, 1991; Cohen *et al.*, 1995; Cohen *et al.*, 1999). Indeed GI microbial ecology is very susceptible to abrupt changes (Goodson *et al.*, 1988; de Fombelle *et al.*, 2001).

Quite recently, an exceptional interest appeared for new nutritional supplements, mainly prebiotics and probiotics for which substantial literature have pointed out the positive impact on the microbial balance in the GIT of different animal species (monogastric animals and ruminants) or in humans for the last decade. Microbial feed additives in diet improve productivity and the effect of yeast culture on volatile fatty acids (VFA) proportion has been widely reported. Inulin-type fructans also enhance the production of VFA within the hindgut and improve the mucosal structure in different animal species. The effects of prebiotics and probiotics, the predominant supplements, have been and are currently investigated on the GI microbial communities in horses.

This paper will present a short review of the gut microorganisms in the adult horse and discuss the effect of various dietary practices on the microflora of the GIT.

Panorama of the gastro-intestinal microflora in adult horses

The abundance, diversity and activity of the microorganisms differ considerably between the gastro-intestinal regions, which offer different environmental conditions to the microflora. The majority of the information available concerns the large intestine and especially the cecum, probably because fitting a cannula on this compartment is relatively easy. The lack of microbiological data are mainly due to the difficulty of collecting digestive content from live and conscious horses. As a consequence, many studies use fecal samples which arises the question about their representativeness of the GI tract microflora. The fecal ecosystem does not represent the foregut ecosystem neither the cecal ecosystem (de Fombelle *et al.*, 2003; Julliand and Goachet, 2005). On the contrary, faeces could be appropriate markers to study the horse colonic ecosystem (Julliand and Goachet, 2005; Da Veiga *et al.*, 2005).

The progress of microscopy and cultural conditions under strictly anaerobiosis (Hungate, 1950) was decisive for isolating and describing intestinal microflora and improving our knowledge on this microflora. However, most microorganisms have yet to be identified. The recent development of culture independent methods and biomolecular based analysis represents a new step in the search for better understanding the microbial diversity of the GI ecosystems.

In the stomach

In the stomach the first individual pocket of the GIT, the average concentrations of total anaerobic bacteria reach 10^9 cfu.ml^{-1} of gastric content (de Fombelle *et al.*, 2003). Populations of lactobacilli, streptococci and lactate-utilizing bacteria are numbered at high level up to 10^8 cfu.ml^{-1} of gastric content (de Fombelle *et al.*, 2003; Alexander and Avies, 1963; Varloud *et al.*, 2004). *Lactobacillus salivarius*, *L. crispatus*, *L. reuteri* and *L. agilis* were identified from the gastric mucosa (Yuki *et al.*, 2000) whereas *L. salivarius*, *L. mucosa*, *L. delbrueckii* were identified from the gastric juice (Al Jassin *et al.*, 2005). These bacteria are mainly involved in the metabolism of starch and highly fermentable carbohydrates, inducing large productions of total lactate concentration *in vitro* (Jassin *et al.*, 2005) and *in vivo*, reaching up to 0.7 g.l^{-1}, 3:30 postprandial (Varloud *et al.*, 2003), and volatile fatty acids. Total VFA concentration approximate 0.4 g.l^{-1} in gastric juice, with a very large proportion of acetate (up to 90%) (Varloud *et al.*, 2003). The gastric microflora probably plays an important role regarding the health of its host via the composition of VFA. Some VFA were indeed reported to be implicated in the pathophysiology of gastric ulcers (Nadeau *et al.*, 2003a, Nadeau *et al.*, 2003b).

The small intestine

The small intestine offers favorable environmental parameters for large densities of strictly anaerobes, ranging from 10^6 to 10^9 cfu.ml^{-1} of intestinal content (de Fombelle *et al.*, 2003; Kern *et al.*, 1974; Mackie and Wilkins, 1988; Kollarczik *et al.*, 1992). Lactobacilli, enterobacteria, enterococci, streptococci, lactate-utilizing bacteria constitute the predominant cultivable microflora. The concentrations of lactobacilli decline from the stomach to the small intestine whereas streptococci counts increase and were reported to be more important in the small intestine than lactobacilli (de Fombelle *et al.*, 2003). The presence of Clostridia sp., Proteus sp., Staphylococci sp., Pseudomonas sp. but also of yeast classified as Candida sp. were reported at a low level in the small intestine: less than 10^3 cfu.ml^{-1} of jejunal content (Kollarczik *et al.*, 1992). The major nutritional function of the microorganisms in the small intestine is the utilization of starch and highly fermentable carbohydrates. Lactate is the major end-product, which concentration decreases constantly from the duodenum to the ileum, and is lower than in the stomach (de Fombelle *et al.*, 2003; Wolter and Chaabouni, 1979).

Although the autochthonous microflora probably contributes directly and indirectly as a barrier in the small intestine, this aspect is not documented in horses.

In the different entities of the hindgut

In the different entities of the hindgut (the cecum, the right and left ventral colon, the left and right dorsal colon, the transverse colon and the descending colon) a large density of strictly anaerobic microorganisms has been reported: concentrations of total anaerobic bacteria vary from 10^7 up to 10^9 cfu.ml^{-1} in the cecum (Julliand *et al.*, 2001; Goodson *et al.*, 1988; de Fombelle *et al.*, 2003; Kern *et al.*, 1974; Mackie and Wilkins, 1988; Kern *et al.*, 1973; Bellet, 1982; Baruc *et al.*,1983; Maczulak *et al.*, 1985; de Vaux and Julliand, 1992; Moore and Dehority, 1993; Julliand *et al.*, 1999; Medina *et al.*, 2002) and are generally lower than in the colon (Julliand *et al.*, 2001; Kern *et al.*, 1974; Mackie and Wilkins, 1988; Moore and Dehority, 1993; Medina *et al.*, 2002); concentration of ciliate protozoa vary from 10^2 to 10^5 cells.ml^{-1} of intestinal content (Goodson *et al.*, 1988; Kern *et al.*, 1974; Kern *et al.*, 1973; Moore and Dehority, 1993); concentration of fungal zoospores vary from 10 to 10^4.ml^{-1} in the cecal content (Orpin, 1981; Julliand, 1996).

Different genera of yeast (Batista *et al.*, 1961), strictly anaerobic fungi (Gold *et al.*, 1988; Li *et al.*, 1989; Gaillard-Martinie *et al.*, 1992; Breton *et al.*, 1991; Li and Heath, 1993; Gaillard-Martinie *et al.*, 1995) and protozoa (Hsiung, 1930; Adam, 1951) have been identified in large intestinal contents. Some bacterial species have been isolated from the hindgut content (Baruc *et al.*,1983; Maczulak *et al.*, 1985; De Vaux *et al.*, 1998) and recently, the biodiversity was studied using molecular tools (Daly and Shirazi-Beechey, 2003).

We will focus on the microorganisms that play major nutritional functions. Average pH values of the hindgut fluctuate around 7, which contributes to provide a favorable environment for the microbial activities. Fungi and bacteria adhering to particles are very largely implicated in the degradation of cell-walls polysaccharides, exhibiting an intense fibrolytic activity. The three main fibre degrading bacteria,

Fibrobacter succinogenes, *Ruminococcus flavefaciens* and *Ruminococcus albus*, have been detected in the intestinal content (Julliand *et al.*, 1999; Bonhomme, 1986; Lin and Stahl, 1995; Drogoul, 2000; Drogoul *et al.*, 2000). Concentrations of cellulolytic bacteria vary between 10^4 and 10^7 per ml of intestinal content (Julliand *et al.*, 2001; Kern *et al.*, 1974; Mackie and Wilkins, 1988; Moore and Dehority, 1993; Medina *et al.*, 2002) and represent a small percentage of the total anaerobes counts in horses (between 0.04% and 9 %) (Kern *et al.*, 1973; Julliand, 1996; Medina, 2003). The proportion of cellulolytics among total anaerobes appeared to be greater in the cecum than in the lower parts of the hindgut, and confirmed that this blind pocket was probably the most propitious for cellulolysis (de Fombelle *et al.*, 2003). High concentrations of VFA are produced, averaging 58 mmol.l^{-1} in the cecal content and 67 mmol.l^{-1} in the colon of animals fed a forage-based diet (Kern *et al.*, 1974; Drogoul, 2000; Drogoul *et al.*, 2000; Hintz *et al.*, 1971; Tisserand *et al.*, 1977; Tisserand *et al.*, 1980; Engelhardt *et al.*, 1992). The main VFA produced are acetate (around 75%), propionate (around 18%) and butyrate (around 6%).

Microorganisms, essentially those adhering to particles, are also responsible for a starch degrading activity in the hindgut, leading to the production of lactate that can average 2 g.l^{-1} (de Fombelle *et al.*, 2001; de Fombelle *et al.*, 2003; Wolter. and Chaabouni, 1979; Medina *et al.*, 2002; Willard *et al.*, 1977; Wolter *et al.*, 1978). The lactate concentration is similar in the cecum and the right ventral colon but increases from the left ventral colon to the left dorsal colon. (de Fombelle *et al.*, 2001; de Fombelle *et al.*, 2003; Medina *et al.*, 2002). Glycolytic and amylolytic bacteria are mainly constituted of streptococci, lactobacilli identified as *Lactobacillus mucosae*, *L. mitsuokella jalaludinii* in the cecum, *L. salivarius* in the (Jassin *et al.*, 2005) and lactate utilizers identified as *Veillonella* sp. and *Megasphaera* sp. (Baruc *et al.*,1983; Maczulak *et al.*, 1985). The average concentrations of streptococci, of lactobacilli and of lactate-utilizing bacteria in the cecum approximate 10^7 cfu.ml^{-1} and are higher in the colon than in the cecum: respectively (Julliand *et al.*, 2001; de Fombelle *et al.*, 2001; de Fombelle *et al.*, 2003; Medina *et al.*, 2002). It appeared that soluble carbohydrates and undigested starch that flowed very quickly through the cecum and entered the colon, could limit their impact on the cecal microflora but enhance it on the colonic microflora (de Fombelle *et al.*, 2001; de Fombelle *et al.*, 2003).

Cecal bacteria show a proteolytic activity *in vitro*, suggesting that cecal bacteria may be capable of contributing to the amino-acid metabolism of the horse (Baruc *et al.*,1983; Maczulak *et al.*, 1985) contrary to urea that may not be used as non-protein nitrogen feed source.

In the hindgut, the local microorganisms maintain the integrity and the balance of the ecosystem, contributing to prevent intestinal disorders and to form a barrier against pathogens. Various stressful conditions, for instance the abrupt change of the diet (Garner *et al.*, 1978; Goodson *et al.*, 1988; de Fombelle *et al.*, 2001) may be responsible for disorders (colic, laminitis, acute colitis, etc), due to the disruption of the normal microflora of the hindgut (Garner *et al.*, 1978; Goodson *et al.*, 1988; de Fombelle *et al.*, 2001). This will be discussed in the next part.

Responses of the gastro-intestinal microflora to dietary treatments in adult horses

This part will focus on the impact of dietary carbohydrates on the GI microflora which is documented whereas the effect of other feed components (dietary proteins, lipids, minerals) remains unknown.

Impact of the diet on the foregut microflora

Despite its probable interest regarding on one hand the nutritional implication and on the other hand the occurrence of gastric ulcer, few studies have been conducted about the impact of nutrition on the gastric ecosystem. The observations conducted on the chyme indicate clearly that meal composition influences the diversity and the activities of the microflora. When horses were fed a high-starch pelleted meal compared to a high-fiber pelleted meal of concentrate, the proportion of lactobacilli and lactate-utilizing bacteria increased in the stomach (de Fombelle *et al.*, 2003). Previous results reported an increase of total VFA and of lactate concentrations in the gastric juice when more energy was supplied to the meal (Nadeau *et al.*, 2000; Nadeau, personal communication).

In the horse stomach, the post-prandial microbial and biochemical kinetics have been recently studied *in vivo* (Varloud *et al.*, 2004) and shows that the concentration of total anaerobes increases rapidly: from about 10^6 to 10^7 during the first hour post-prandial and up to 10^8 cfu.ml^{-1}

gastric juice after 3:30 hours. Lactobacilli and Streptococci counts also increase from 10^5 to 10^6 within the first hour and up to 10^7 cfu.ml^{-1} after 3:30 hours. The concentration of lactate-utilizing bacteria increases in a lower proportion and reaches around 10^5 cfu.ml^{-1} gastric juice after 3:30 post-prandial. This is consistent with the measurements of end-products: Lactate concentration increases from 0.1 to 0.2, 0.3, 0.7 g.l^{-1}, 1:00, 2:00, 3:30 after the meal. During the 3:30 hours following the meal, total VFA increases from 0.1 to 0.4 g.l^{-1}, where acetate represents 60 %.

The addition of starch in the meal has an impact on the bacterial jejunal counts: barley, maize and amylase, maize and soybean meal are the best promoters of total anaerobes and *Lactobacilli* sp. (Kollarczik *et al.*, 1992). An increase of the concentration of lactobacilli, as well as those of streptococci and lactate-utilizers was also reported in the ileum of horses fed a high-starch pelleted meal compared to a high-fiber pelleted meal of concentrate (de Fombelle *et al.*, 2003).

Impact of the diet on the hindgut microflora

Both the profiles and the activities of the microflora in the hindgut of horses are sensitive to the forage/concentrate ratio of the diet and especially to the relative quantity of starch. Increasing the quantity of starch in a meal exceeds the capacity of the small intestine to digest starch and allows a greater amount of non-degraded starch to reach the hindgut (Potter *et al.*, 1992; Kienzle, 1994). Starch is then available for the local microflora and microfauna. In the colon, the protozoal counts increase slightly when concentrate is added (Moore and Dehority, 1993) and the proportion of holotrichs increases both in the cecum and colon (Kern *et al.*, 1973; Moore and Dehority, 1993).

Starch induces an increase of the total anaerobes counts in the cecum (Julliand *et al.*, 2001; de Fombelle *et al.*, 2003; Medina *et al.*, 2002) and in the right ventral colon (Julliand *et al.*, 2001; de Fombelle *et al.*, 2003; Bellet, 1982; Moore and Dehority, 1993; Medina *et al.*, 2002). The concentration of lactobacilli and streptococci is also increased (Garner *et al.*, 1978; Goodson *et al.*, 1988; Medina, 2003) in the intestinal contents. The increase of lactate-utilizing bacteria remains inferior to lactate-producing bacteria (Julliand *et al.*, 2001; Medina, 2003). As a consequence, the concentration of lactic acid is enhanced while pH decreases with a minimal value appearing 5 h after feeding, in the

Véronique Julliand

hindgut. And cecal concentration of cellulolytic bacteria decreases 4 h after feeding (Julliand *et al.*, 2001; Garner *et al.*, 1978; Medina, 2003), inducing a significant decrease of the [(acetate + butyrate) / propionate] ratio, which suggests a decline in the fibrolytic activity.

Several authors have reported that disturbances due to the fermentation of starch in the hindgut can lead to changes in the microbial activities as well as the environmental parameters and finally provoke pathologies. Mungall *et al.*, 2001 suggested that the rapid increase of *Streptococci* sp. in the caecum and colon observed in parallel with carbohydrate overload may directly cause laminitis via production of endotoxin(s) capable of activating MMPs (matrix metallo-proteinases) within lamellar structure of the hoof.

A strategy to limit the negative consequences of cereal-based diets on the equine intestinal ecosystem is to increase digestion of starch in the small intestine (Kienzle, 1994). Thermal processes of starch can thus be beneficial. Another strategy is to maintain a high ratio forage/concentrate in the ration which means adding rather than substituting concentrate to forage. Regarding cellulolytic bacteria, their concentration increases when the proportion of concentrate increases from zero to 30% in the cecum and right ventral colon (Julliand *et al.*, 2001; Kern *et al.*, 1973; Bellet, 1982; de Vaux and Julliand, 1992; Julliand, 1996) and also in the left dorsal colon (de Fombelle *et al.*, 2003). On the opposite side, when the proportion of concentrate goes over 50% of the total ration, the density of cellulolytic bacteria declines severely (Julliand *et al.*, 2001).

Impact of an abrupt change of the diet on the GI microflora

The sudden incorporation of concentrate in the ration provokes an increase of the total anaerobes counts in the cecum (Goodson *et al.*, 1988; de Fombelle *et al.*, 2001) and in the right ventral colon (de Fombelle *et al.*, 2001). In parallel of this increase, a change in the profile of bacterial populations is noticed, much more important when the percentage of concentrate is high in the total ration (Garner *et al.*, 1978; de Fombelle *et al.*, 2001).

To prevent the negative impact of a sudden change of the diet, new feeds must be incorporated gradually in the ration.

Responses of the gastro-intestinal microflora to pre- and pro-biotics in adult horses

The use of pre- or probiotics has been proposed to manipulate the environment and the microbial activities of the intestinal ecosystem in order to limit the negative consequences of cereal-based diets on the equine intestinal ecosystem.

Prebiotics

Prebiotic compounds have firstly been defined as *non digestible food ingredients that beneficially affect the host by selectively stimulating the growth and/or activity of one or a limited number of bacterial species already present in the colon* (Gibson and Roberfroid, 1995). An updated definition that extends the effect of prebiotics to the whole digestive tract is now accepted: *selectively fermented ingredients that allow specific changes, both in the composition and/or activity in the gastrointestinal microflora that confers benefits upon host wellbeing and health* (Gibson et al., 2004). Prebiotics selectively increase the numbers of lactic acid bacteria, and especially *Lactobacilli* sp. and *Bifidobacteria* sp., to the detriment of potential pathogenic bacteria such as *Clostridium* spp. Inulin-type fructans (β(2-1)fructans) such as inulin and oligofructose also named fructo-oligosaccharide (FOS), lactulose and transgalacto-oligosaccharides (TOS) are the three oligosaccharides with demonstrated prebiotic properties (Gibson et al., 2004). Literature about the action of prebiotics on the equine GI microflora is very scarce.

Wolter (1999) observed a decrease of colic incidence in a population of 126 horses supplemented with oligofructose (β(2-1)fructans with degree of polymerisation DP ranging from 3 to 7, average DP = 4) and noticed a strong decrease of putrefactive compounds in their feces. An experiment conducted on 40 horses receiving increasing levels of oligofructose or lactulose in their diet confirmed the decrease of the incidence of colic and showed a proportional effect to the quantity of supplemented prebiotics (Orafti, personal communication).

Changes of the microflora due to the supplementation of oligofructose in the diets appear in the feces (Pellegrini et al., 1999; Berg et al., 2005): counts of lactobacilli do not change while *E. coli* level decrease; pH decreases whereas lactate and SCFA (acetate, propionate and butyrate) concentrations increase in the fecal content (Berg *et al.*, 2005). Interestingly, Respondek *et al.*, 2005 measured modifications in the stomach and in the right ventral colon of horses receiving oligofructose. Counts of total bacteria, streptococci and lactate-utilising bacteria increased in the gastric juice and the pH was higher when oligofructose was supplemented, which may contribute to diminish the risk of gastric ulcers (Nadeau *et al.*, 2000). Detailed data are reported in the present ENUCO Scientific.

Probiotics

The term probiotics (literally *for life*) was proposed in opposition to antibiotics (*against life*). Probiotics are defined as *living microbial preparations that have a beneficial action for the host by improving digestion and intestinal hygiene.* They are also known as digestive bioregulators or direct-fed microbials. Today a large range of defined strains of probiotics belong to the group of lactic acid bacteria (*Bifidobacteria, Lactobacillus, Streptococcus, Enterococcus* and *Lactococcus* species), *Bacillus* sp., fungi (*Aspergillus* sp.) and yeasts (*Saccharomyces* sp.). Few scientific studies have been conducted to demonstrate the action of probiotics on the equine GI microflora.

Lactic acid bacteria and Bacillus sp.

A study showed that a daily supplementation, during 5 weeks, of 10^{10} spores of *Bacillus cereus*, strain BCIP5832, induced an increase of total anaerobic and proteolytic bacteria in the cecum (de Vaux and Julliand, 1992).

Recently a variety of lactobacilli, either host-specific or not, have been evaluated as potential probiotics (Weese *et al.*, 2003; Weese *et al.*, 2004). Intestinal colonization of *Lactobacillus rhamnosus* strain GG, supplemented for 5 days at doses of 10^9, 10^{10} or 5.10^{10} cfu.50 kg^{-1} bodyweight.day^{-1}, is sporadic and poor (Weese *et al.*, 2003). On the other hand, *L. pensosus* strain WE7, isolated from equine fecal samples, was recovered from the faeces after an oral administration. This strain was inhibitory *in vitro* against *Escherichia coli*, *Salmonella zooepidemicus*, *Clostridium difficile* and mildly against *Clostridium perfringens* (Weese *et al.*, 2004).

Fungi and yeast

The effect of *Aspergillus oryzae* has been evaluated *in vitro* on equine cecal fermentation. The addition of *Aspergillus oryzae* resulted in little change at the current recommended levels but improved fibrolytic activity at 10 times (McDaniel *et al.*, 1993).

Most studies on probiotics in equine were conducted with *Saccharomyces cerevisiae* (SC). Zootechnical effects such as the improvement of milk quality in mares or of growth in foals, have been demonstrated (Glade, 1991c; Glade, 1991d). The impact of SC on digestibility has been reported in about fifteen articles (Medina, 2003; Glade and Biesik, 1986; Glade and Sist, 1988; Pagan, 1990; Hall *et al.*, 1990; Glade, 1991a; Glade, 1991b; Glade, 1991[e]; Kim *et al.*, 1991; Glade, 1992; Hausenblasz *et al.*, 1993; Moore *et al.*, 1994; Hill and Gutsell, 1998). Data vary according to the strain of *Saccharomyces cerevisiae*, the quantity supplemented to the horse and the composition of the ration. Interestingly, the positive effect of SC supplementation on total cell-wall fibre (NDF) digestibility decreases when the proportion of concentrate increases in the ration. An increase in the digestibility of phosphorus indicated also a positive effect of SC on cecal fermentation (Pagan, 1990).

SC are able to reach and survive in the cecum and to a lesser extent in the right ventral colon of horses supplemented daily, but not to colonize them (Medina, 2003; Moore *et al.*, 1994). Supplementing SC, especially to cereal-rich diets, enhances the overall pH values and reduces the post-prandial decrease in the cecum and the colon (Medina, 2003; Moore *et al.*, 1994). This is closely related to the decrease of lactic acid concentration, in combination with a decrease in the lactic acid-utilizing to lactic acid-producing bacteria ratio (Medina, 2003). The exact role of SC in reducing lactate production in the hindgut and on stabilizing the cecal environment is not clear but it is likely that similar modes of action to those in the rumen of the cow are present in the hindgut of the horse. The molar percentage of acetate increases in the cecum and the colon with SC supplementation, in correlation with an enhancement of cellulolytics counts (Moore *et al.*, 1994) or of the fibrolytic activity (Medina, 2003).

These observations suggest that yeast supplementation may allow some horses to better tolerate high starch diets without developing digestive disorders.

Many investigations have been conducted, principally in hamsters, rats and mice, on the effect of *Saccharomyces cerevisiae* (or *S. boulardii*) on *Clostridium difficile* infection. Yeast shows beneficial effects that would be of particular interest in horses.

Conclusion and perspectives

It is beyond doubt that nutrition interacts with the gastro-intestinal microflora in horses which justifies the special care that must be taken in the management of feeding. Practically, to prevent alterations of the GI ecosystem, attention has to be paid first on feeding practices. Horse keepers should respect the regularity of the ration, in term of nature and daily distribution, and carefully adapt the diet to the exercise level. They should also respect nutritional transition of 4 to 8 days each time there is a change: change of feeds, change of feed batch, change to pasture, return to box, etc.

Concerning the use of pre- and probiotics, the first results are encouraging and more studies are certainly required to deeply understand the direct effects of these nutritional supplements on the GI microflora in the horse. Prebiotic feed ingredients were shown to better balance microbial fermentation into various short chain fatty acids (with emphasis on butyrate production), which results in improved intestinal barrier function. Probiotics improve nutrition through their impact on digestive processes and especially on the GI microflora. During their passage through the intestinal tract, they exert particular effects on digestive processes (e.g. interactions with mucosal immune system) and they potentially prevent the development of pathogens. Through their action, both pre- and probiotics contribute to the animal welfare.

There are interesting possibilities to combine the use of prebiotics and probiotics because their actions are complementary:
- Pre- and probiotics can be used as synbiotics: prebiotics can decrease the lag-time of the probiotics, which enhances the impact of the microorganisms in the gastro-intestinal tract.

- Pre- and probiotics can be used simultaneously considering that both affect similar physiological processes (immunology, zootechnical performance, improved bowel habit), but via different and independent pathways.

Some limitations in our knowledge are linked to the lack of information about the understanding of the microbial diversity of the GI tract. Also the representativeness of fecal samples is uncertain although most studies use feces as marker of the GI tract microflora. The current development of biomolecular based analysis complementary to classical microbial techniques will enlighten our comprehension of the GI ecosystem.

References

Adam, K.M.G., 1951. The quantity and distribution of the ciliate protozoa in the large in testine of the horse. Parasitology;41:301-311.

Al Jassin, R.A.M., Scott P.T., Trebbin A.L., *et al.*, 2005. The genetic diversity of lactic acid producing bacteria in the equine gastrointestinal tract. FEMS Microbiology Letters 248:75-81.

Alexander, F. and Davies E., 1963. Production and fermentation of lactate by bacteria in the alimentary canal of the horse and pig. J. Comp. Path.;73:1-8.

Baruc, C.J., Dawson, K.A. and Baker, J.P., 1983. The caracterization and nitrogen metabolism of equine caecal bacteria. 8th ENPS;151-156.

Batista, A., Chaves, U., Cte de Vasconcelos, *et al.*, 1961. Flora micoteca intestinal de equinos e asininos no recife. Inst. Micol. Univ. Recife;326:116.

Bellet, S., 1982. Etude des effets de différents régimes sur la microflore cæcale et colique de poney. ED des Sciences de la vie et de la Santé. Dijon: Université de Bourgogne;121.

Berg, E.L., Fu, C.J., Porter, J.H., *et al.*, 2005. Fructooligosaccharide supplementation in the yearling horse : effects on fecal pH, microbial content, and volatile fatty acid concentrations. J. Anim. Sci. ;83:1549-1553.

Bonhomme, A., 1986. Attachment of horse cecal bacteria to forage cell walls. J. Vet. Sci.;48:313-322.

Breton, A., Dusser, M., Gailliard-Martinie, B., *et al.*, 1991. *Piromyces rhizinflata* nov. sp., a stritly anaerobic fungus from faeces of the saharian ass: a morphological, metabolic and ultrastructural study. FEMS Microbiol. lett.;82:1-8.

Cohen, N., Matejka, P.L., Honnas, C.M., *et al.*, 1995. Case-control study of the association between various management factors and development of colic in horses. Journal of American Veterinary Medical Association;206:667-673.

Cohen, N.D., Gibbs, P.G. and Woods, A.M., 1999. Dietary and other management factors associated with colic in horses. Journal of American Veterinary Medical Association 215:53-60.

Da Veiga, L., Chaucheyras-Durand, F. and Julliand, V., 2005. Comparative study of colon and faeces microbial communities and activities in horses fed a high starch diet. 3rd European Conference on Horse Nutrition.

Daly, K. and Shirazi-Beechey, S.P., 2003. Design and evaluation of group-specific oligonucleotide probes for quantitative analysis of intestinal ecosystems : their application to assessment of equine colonic microflora. FEMS Microbiology Ecology;44:243-252.

de Fombelle, A., Julliand, V., Drogoul, C., et al., 2001. Feeding and microbial disorders in horses : 1-effects of an abrupt incorporation of two levels of barley in a hay diet on microbial profile and activities. Journal of Equine Veterinary Science;21:439-445.

de Fombelle, A., Varloud, M., Goachet, A.-G., et al., 2003. Characterisation of the microbial and biochemical profile of the different segments of the digestive tract in horses fed two distinct diets. Animal Science;77:293-304.

de Vaux, A. and Julliand, V., 1992. Effet d'un probiotique sur la flore bacterienne et la biochimie du caecum chez le poney. 20ème réunion de l'association française pour la gnotoxémie, 17 décembre.

de Vaux, A., Laguerre, G., Diviès, C., et al., 1998. Enterococcus asini sp. nov. isolated from the caecum of donkeys (Equus asinus). International Journal of Systematic Bacteriology 48:383-387.

Drogoul, C., 2000. Influence de la granulométrie du fourrage sur la digestin des parois végétales chez le poney en relation avec les modifications du transit et de l'activité fibrolytique des écosystèmes caecal et colique. Ecole Doctorale des sciences de la Vie et de la Santé. Dijon: Université de Bourgogne 167.

Drogoul, C., Poncet, C. and Tisserand, J.L., 2000. Feeding ground and pelleted hay rather than chopped hay to ponies. 2: Consequences on fibre degradation in the cecum and the colon. Animal feed science and technology 87:131-145.

Engelhardt, W.V., Burmester, M., Hansen, K., et al., 1992. Transepithelialer transport von acetat, propionat und butyrat im ceacum, im proximalen und im distalen colon von ponys. 1. Europäische Konferenz über die Ernährung des pferdes. Physiologie und Pathologie des Verdauungskanals - Konsequenzen für die Ernährung, p. 171-174.

Gaillard-Martinie, B., Breton, A., Dusser, M., et al., 1992. Contribution to the morphological, cytological and ultrastructural characterization of Piromyces mae, a strictly anaerobic rumen fungus. Curr. Microbiol.;24:159-164.

Gaillard-Martinie, B., Breton, A., Dusser, M., *et al.*, 1995. *Piromyces citronii* sp. nov., a stricly anaerobic fungus from the equine caecum: a morphological, metabolic and ultrastructural study. FEMS Microbiol. Lett. 130:321-326.

Garner, H.E., Moore, J.N., Johnson, J.H., *et al.*, 1978. Changes in the caecal flora associated with the onset of laminitis. Equine Veterinary Journal 10:249-252.

Gibson, G.R. and Roberfroid, M.B., 1995. Dietary modulation of the human colonic microbiota: introducing the concept of prebiotics. J. Nutri. 125:1401-1412.

Gibson, G.R., Probert, H., Van Loo, J., *et al.*, 2004. Dietary modulation of the human colonic microbiota : uptating the concept of prebiotics. Nutr. Res. Rev. 17:259-275.

Glade, M.J. and Biesik, L.M., 1986 Enhanced nitrogen retention in yearling horses supplemented with yeast culture. Journal of Animal Science 62:1635-1640.

Glade, M.J. and Sist, M.D., 1988 Dietary yeast cultures supplementation enhances urea recycling in the equine large intestine. Nutrition Reports International 37:11-17.

Glade, M.J., 1991a. Effects of dietary yeast culture supplementation of mares explored. Feedstuffs 15.

Glade, M.J., 1991b. Dietary yeast culture supplementation of mares during late gestation and early lactation: effects on dietary nutrient digestibilities and fecal nitrogen partitioning. Journal of Equine Veterinary Science 11:10-16.

Glade, M.J., 1991c. Dietary yeast culture supplementation of mares during late gestation and early lactation: effects on milk production, milk composition, weight gain and linear growth of nursing foals. Journal of Equine Veterinary Science 11:89-95.

Glade, M.J., 1991d. Dietary yeast culture supplementation of mares during late gestation and early lactation: effects on mare and foal plasma metabolite, amino acide and endocrine profiles. Journal of Equine Veterinary Science 11:167-175.

Glade, M.J., 1991e. Effects of dietary yeast culture supplementation of lactating mares on the digestibility and retention of the nutrient delivered to nursing foals via milk. Journal of Equine Veterinary Science 11:323-329.

Glade, M.J., 1992. Viable yeast culture in equine nutrition. Supplement to proceedings of Alltech's eighth annual symposium:1-26.

Gold, J.J., Heath, I.B. and Bauchop, T., 1988. Ultrastructural description of a new chytrid genus of caecum anaerobe *Caecomyces equi* gen. nov., sp. nov., assigned to the Neocallimasticaecceae. BioSystems 21:403-415.

Goodson, J., Tyznik, W.J., Cline, J.H., *et al.*, 1988. Effects of an abrupt diet change from hay to concentrate on microbial numbers and physical environment in the cecum of the pony. Applied and Environmental Microbiology 54:1946-1950.

Hall, R.R., Jackson, S.G., Baker, J.P., *et al.*, 1990. Influence of yeast culture supplementation on ration digestion by horses. Journal of Equine Veterinary Science 10:130-134.

Hausenblasz, J., Szuco, J. and Mezes M., 1993. Effect of viable yeast culture supplementation on nutrient digestibility and feed utilization of growing cold-blooded horses. 9th Biotechnology in the Feed Industry symposium;Poster.

Hill, J. and Gutsell, S., 1998. Effect of supplementation of a hay and concentrate diet with live yeast culture on the digestibility of nutrients in 2 and 3 year old riding school horses. BSAS annual meeting, p.128.

Hintz, H.F., Argenzio, R.A. and Schryver, H.F., 1971. Digestion coefficients, blood glucose levels and molar percentage of volatile acids in intestinal fluid of ponies fed varying forage-grain ratios. Journal of Animal Science 33:992-995.

Hsiung, T.S., 1930. A monograph of the protozoa of the large intestine of the horse. Iowa Stage. Coll. J. Sci. 4:356-423.

Hudson, J.M., Cohen, N.D., Gibbs, P.G., *et al.*, 2001. Feeding practices associated with colic in horses. Journal of American Veterinary Medical Association 219:1419-1425.

Hungate, R.E., 1950. The anaerobic mesophilic cellulolytic bacteria. *Bacteriol. Rev.* 14:1-46.

Julliand, V. and Goachet, A.-G., 2005. Fecal microflora as a marker of cecal or colonic microflora in horses? 19th Symposium p.140-141.

Julliand, V., 1996. Etude de l'écosystème cæcal des équidés : aptitude à dégrader les polyolosides pariétaux, Caractérisation quantitative et qualitative des flores cellulolytiques bactériennes et fongiques dominantes. ENSBANA. Dijon: Université de bourgogne, p.121.

Julliand, V., de Fombelle, A., Drogoul, C., *et al.*, 2001. Feeding and microbial disorders in horses: 3-Effects of three hay:grain ratios on microbial profile and activities. Journal of Equine Veterinary Science 21:543-546.

Julliand, V., de Vaux, A., Millet, L., *et al.*, 1999. Identification of *Ruminococcus flavefaciens* as the Predominant cellulolytic bacterial species of the equine cecum. Applied Environmental Microbiology 65:3738-3741.

Kern, D.L., Slyter, L.L., Leffel, E.C., *et al.*, 1974. Ponies vs.steers: microbial and chemical characteristics of intestinal ingesta. Journal of Animal Science 38:559-564.

Kern, D.L., Slyter, L.L., Weaver, J.M., *et al.*, 1973. Pony cecum *vs.* steer rumen : the effect of oats and hay on the microbial ecosystem. Journal of Animal Science 37:463-469.

Kienzle, E., 1994. Small intestinal digestion of starch in the horse. Revue de médecine vétérinaire 145:199-204.

Kim, S.M., Kim, C.M., Lee, H.K., *et al.*, 1991. Evaluation of nutrients values of some feedstuffs, and the effects of yeast culture supplementation on digestibilities of nutrients and blood parameter in horse. Korean Journal of Animal Nutrition and feedstuff 15:272-280.

Kollarczik, B., Enders, C., Friedrich, M., *et al.*, 1992. Auswirkungen der rationszusammensetzung auf das keimsperktrum im jejunum von pferden. 1. Europäische Konferenz über die Ernährung des pferdes. Physiologie und Pathologie des Verdauungskanals - Konsequenzen für die Ernährung;49-54.

Li, J. and Heath, I.B., 1993. Chytridiomycetous gut fungi, oft overlooked contributors to herbivore digestion. Can. J. Microbiol. 39:1003-1013.

Li, J., Heath, I.B. and Bauchop, T., 1989. *Piromyces mae* and *Piromyces dumbonica*, two new species of uniflagellate anaerobic chytridiomycete fungi from the hindgut of the horse and elephant. Canadian Journal of Botanic 68:1021-1033.

Lin, C. and Stahl, D.A., 1995. Taxon-specific probes for the cellulolytic genus *Fibrobacter* reveal abundant and novel equine-associated population. Applied Environmental Microbiology 61:1348-1351.

Mackie, R.I. and Wilkins, C.A., 1988. Enumeration of anaerobic bacterial microflora of the equine gastrointestinal tract. Applied Environmental Microbiology 54:2155-2160.

Maczulak, A.E., Dawson, K.A. and Baker, J.P., 1985. Nitrogen utilisation in bacterial isolates from the equine cæcum. Applied Environmental Microbiology 50:1439-1443.

McDaniel, A.L., Martin, S.A., MsCann, J.S., *et al.*, 1993. Effects of *Aspergillum oryzae* fermentation extract on *in vitro* equine cecal fermentation. Journal of Animal Science 71:2164-2172.

Medina B., 2003. Effets de la culture de levures vivantes Yea SaccR1026 (CBS 493.94), en fonction de deux ratios luzerne/orge dans un aliment complet granulé, sur le fonctionnement de l'écosystème intestinal du cheval. Dijon, France: Université de Bourgogne,159.

Medina, M., Girard, I.D., Jacotot, E., *et al.*, 2002. Effect of a preparation of *Saccharomyces cerevisiae* on microbial profiles and fermentation patterns in the large intestine of horses fed a high fiber or a high starch diet. Journal of Animal Science 80:2600-2609.

Moore, B.E. and Dehority, B.A., 1993. Effects of diet and hindgut defaunation on diet digestibility and microbial concentrations in the cecum and colon of the horse. Journal of Animal Science 71:3350-3358.

Moore, B.E., Newman, K.E., Spring, P., *et al.*, 1994. Effect of yeast culture (Yea Sacc 1026) on microbial populations and digestion in the cecum and colon of the equine. Journal of Animal Science 72:252.

Mungall, B.A., Kyaw-Tanner, M. and Politt, C.C., 2001. In vitro evidence for a bacterial pathogenesis of equine laminitis. Veterinary Microbiology 79:209-223.

Nadeau, J.A., Andrews, F.M., Mathew, A.G., *et al.*, 2000. Evaluation of diet as a cause of gastric ulcers in horses. American Journal of Veterinary Research 61:784-790.

Orpin, C.G., 1981. Isolation of cellulolytic phycomycete fungi from the cæcum of the horse. Journal of Generic Microbiology 123:287-296.

Pagan, J.D., 1990. Effect of yeast culture supplementation on nutrient digestibility on mature horses. Journal of Animal Science 68:371.

Pellegrini, L., Miliani, A. and Bergero, D., 1999. Frutto-oligosaccaridi sulla microflora intestinale del cavallo sportivo : nota pratica. Riv. Zoot. Vet. 27:49-51.

Potter, G.D., Arnold, F.F., Householder, D.D., *et al.*, 1992. Digestion of starch in the small or large intestine of the equine. 1. Europäiscche Konferenz über die Ernährung des Pferdes. Physiologie und Pathologie des Verdauungskanals - Konsequenzen für die Ernährung 107-111.

Proudman, C.J., 1991. A two years survey of equine colic in general practice. *Equine* Veterinary Journal 24:90-93.

Reeves, M.J., Salman, M.D. and Smith, G., 1996. Risk factors for equine acute abdominal disease (colic) : results from a multi-center case-control study. Preventive Veterinary Medicine 26:285-301.

Tinker, M., White, N.A., Lessard, P., *et al.*, 1997. Prospective study of equine colic risk factors. Equine Veterinary Journal 29:454-458.

Tisserand, J.L., Masson, C., Ottin-Pecchio, M., *et al.*, 1977. Mesure du pH et de la concentration en AGV dans le caecum et le côlon du poney. Annales de biologie animale, biochimie et biophysique 17:553-557.

Tisserand, J.-L., Ottin-Pechio, M. and Rollin, G., 1980. Effet du mode de distribution du foin et des céréales sur l'activité cellulolytique dans le gros intestin du poney. Reproduction, Nutrition et Développement 20:1685-1689.

Varloud, M., Goachet, A.-G., de Fombelle, A., *et al.*, 2003. Effect of the diet on prececal digestibility of the dietary starch measured on horses. 18th Equine Nutrition and Physiology Symposium.

Varloud, M., Jacotot, E., Fonty, G., *et al.*, 2004. Postprandial evolution of the microbial community and biochemical composition of stomach contents in equines. Reproduction nutrition development 44:S75.

Weese, J.S., Anderson, M.E., Lowe, A., *et al.*, 2004. Screening of the equine intestinal microflora for potential probiotic organisms. Equine veterinary Journal 36:351-355.

Weese, S.J., Anderson, M.E., Lowe, A., *et al.*, 2003. Preliminary investigation of the probiotic potential of lactobacillus rhamnosus strain GG in horses : fecal recovery following oral administration and safety. Canadian Vet. J. 44:299-302.

Willard, J.G., Willard, J.C., Wolfram, S.A., *et al.*, 1977. Effect of diet on cecal pH and feeding behavior of horses. Journal of Animal Science 45:87-93.

Wolter, R. and Chaabouni, A., 1979. Etude de la digestion de l'amidon chez le cheval par analyse du contenu digestif après abattage. Revue de Médecine Vétérinaire 130:1345-1357.

Wolter, R., 1999. Alimentation du cheval. France Agricole Paris:415.

Wolter, R., Gouy, D., Durix, A., *et al.*, 1978. Digestibilité et activité biochimique intracaecale chez le poney recevant un même aliment complet présenté sous forme granulée, expansée ou semi-expansée. Annales de Zootechnie 27:47-60.

Yuki, N., Shimazaki, T., Kushiro, A., *et al.*, 2000. Colonization of the stratified squamous epithelium of the nonsecreting area of horse stomach by lactobacilli. Appl Environ Microbiol 66:5030-5034.

Nutritional management of horses with hoof diseases

Susan A. Kempson
Department of Veterinary Biomedical Sciences, Royal (Dick) School of Veterinary Studies, University of Edinburgh, Summerhall, Edinburgh EH8 9QH, United Kingdom.

Introduction

The keratinized, exterior hoof capsules protect the underlying structures from the external environment. This includes protection from both physical and chemical insult. Transfer of the horse's weight, via the bony column to the ground occurs through the hoof capsule. It is also responsible for much of the shock absorption of movement. Breakdown in the structure of the hoof capsule compromises its functional integrity which leads to lameness, loss of performance and distress to both horse and owner. Hoof diseases will frequently affect all four feet, so lameness is often subtle, particularly in the early stages of the problem. The early indication of foot discomfort or pain are a reluctance to jump, fading towards the end of a marathon, race or cross-country, or a shortening of the stride, particularly on hard ground.

Modern performance horses are larger and heavier than their wild ancestors. However, the feet of today's top show-jumpers, eventers and dressage horses are no bigger than that of the wild Prewejski horse of 14.2 hh. A larger horse, carrying a rider and performing extreme athletic movement is being carried on a relatively small structure. The hoof capsule of the modern horse is close to its mechanical limits. It is no surprise, therefore, that small changes in structure will have a profound effect on function.

In the early 1980s, very few people accepted that nutrition could influence the structure and functional integrity of the equine hoof horn. However, the hoof capsule and its supporting structures, epidermis and dermis, is a highly specialised region of the skin. Nutrition will influence the skin and hair coat and also the hoof horn. The first indication of the importance of nutrition in horn structure came from studies of biotin fed to pigs. Biotin was then fed to horses. Dr Frank Gravlee, studying the blood biochemistry of thoroughbred horses, found that hoof defects were due to lack of a combination of nutrients. From this work in the early 1980s a multinutrient supplement specifically targeted at the hoof horn was developed. By the early 1990s it was recognised that dietary supplements designed to correct poor quality horn were successful.

Today's horses and ponies are now fed highly unnatural diets and are more likely to have hoof disease as a result of dietary excesses of certain nutrients rather than deficiencies.

In order to understand how nutrition affects the hoof horn, an understanding of the structure is essential.

Structure and growth

The equine hoof capsule is the end product of keratinization of the epidermis covering the soft tissues of the foot. Just as in the skin, daughter cells are produced by mitosis in the stratum basale. These daughter cells, the keratinocytes, then undergo maturation, producing keratin proteins and inter-filamentous matrix, which are retained within the cells. The keratinocytes also secrete lipids into the intercellular spaces as they mature towards the stratum corneum. The intercellular lipids are essential for the cell to cell attachment. They also provide the permeability barrier which controls the movement of water across the horn. Lysosomal enzymes are also present within the intercellular lipids which prevent the entry of micro-organisms into the horn.

As the keratinocytes reach the end of the process of keratinisation, their cell organelles are broken down. The keratinocytes become the horn cells or squames of the stratum corneum, also known as the horn. Horn consists of mature keratinocytes, containing keratin fibres and matrix attached to each other by intercellular lipids.

The arrangement and proportions of the keratin fibres to matrix vary from region to region in response to the functional requirements. Intercellular lipids also differ in the various regions, in both quantity and chemistry.

At the junction of the epidermis to the dermis lies the basement membrane. This is a semi-permeable membrane responsible for controlling the passage of nutrients from the underlying dermis. The basement membrane also mediates the attachment of the epidermis and horn to the underlying structures.

The dermis, or corium, contains the blood vessels and nerves as well as the collage and elastic fibres which provide attachment and mechanical support. The epidermis and hoof horn are only as healthy as the underlying dermis (corium). When there is a severe breakdown in the normal function of the dermis, as in laminitis, the consequences for the horn and the horse are very serious.

In order to understand how to manage hoof diseases, the effect of certain nutrients on the structures of the hoof horn will be discussed.

The biotin story

Biotin is one of the B group of vitamins and the first nutrient to be fed to horses with the specific aim of improving the quality of the hoof horn. Horses manufacture biotin in the hind gut and very few horses are biotin deficient, consequently, feeding biotin produced only limited results. Only horses which are highly stressed by work or starvation will show signs of biotin deficiency. Occasionally the same thing will occur in horses which have been receiving long-term antibiotic therapy. Recently, the author has see biotin deficiency in horses receiving pre- and pro-biotics. These supplements are highly detrimental to the intestinal bacteria which produce biotin. A horse with biotin deficiency will show destruction of the horn tubules in the outer layer of the dorsal wall, particularly in the quarles. If the feet are white, there will be bleeding into the horn, particularly in the medial and lateral walls. These horses will respond to biotin supplementation. Biotin deficiency causes a loss of mitosis in the stratum basale. Consequently the tips of the dermal papillae in the coronary region are susceptible to physical trauma which results in haemorrhage from the blood capillaries. The defects in the outer horn tubules can be detected with a magnifying glass. It is important to distinguish the haemorrhage due to biotin deficiency, which starts at the coronary band, from that due to laminitis. Laminitic haemorrhage occurs at the level of the nail holes. These horses will also show a dull hair coat and, if it persists, will go on to develop laminitis.

Calcium

Calcium was the second nutrient to be identified as being significant in hoof horn quality. The traditional equine diet in the United Kingdom was based on hay with feeds of oats, brand and pelletted feed stuff. This diet contained high quantities of phosphorus as phytate, which blocked the absorption of calcium from the intestines.

In the hoof horn, calcium is important for maintaining cell-to-cell (squame to squame) attachment. A deficiency of calcium will cause a crumbling of the hoof horn, particularly around the nail holes and general collapse of the heel horn. Calcium is also necessary for the deposition of the intercellular lipids or fats. If calcium is low in the diet, the horn will also become drier in the summer and more water-logged in the winter. A good course of calcium is alfalfa, as it is protein-bound and more readily absorbed by the horse. Some individuals do have difficulty absorbing calcium from the diet, but can manage well on alfalfa. The ratio of calcium to phosphorus in the diet needs to be 1:6:1, or 2:1 calcium to phosphorus. A good balance is essential.

A deficiency of calcium will lead to inadequate deposition and formation of intercellular lipids. This makes it easy for bacteria in the environment to invade the horn. The pioneer organisms are usually sulphur-reducing bacteria. These are then followed by opportunistic bacteria and fungi. The problem for the horse then becomes more than just a simple dietary one. Numbers of bacteria and fungi must be reduced in order for dietary changes to be effective.

Selenium

Trace minerals act primarily as catalysts or activators in enzymal or hormone systems. Selenium is essential for normal muscle development but as little as 5 parts per million can be toxic for horses. Sheep and cattle have a much higher requirement and tolerance of selenium. Excess of any of the trace minerals may be detrimental. Since feeding supplementary selenium has become fashionable, more and more horses with poor quality horn are showing signs of selenium toxicity.
Selenium substitutes for sulphur in the keratin fibres and the horn cells become weak with little or no mechanical strength. Excess selenium also makes the horn particularly susceptible to bacterial infection, white

line disease and thrush. Horses with persistent thrush, which does not respond to normal treatments, will have low grade selenium toxicity. The frog horn is the fastest growing horn and the selenium salts will be deposited in the horn.

The greatest degree of keratin fibre production occurs at the coronary band and this is the region most affected by excess selenium. Toxicity shows as horizontal cracks in the hooves. In more severe toxicity, there will be a severe coronitis which will become infected and eventually laminitis.

Many factors, including soils, plants environment, age, breed, conditioning and athletic performance can affect trace mineral requirements in horses. Unless a deficiency of selenium has been identified it is best to avoid adding selenium to the diet.

Methionine

Amino acids are the building blocks of proteins. Some amino acids are synthesized within the body from other compounds. Others cannot be manufactured by the animal in sufficient quantity and are the "essential amino acids". Horses require dietary sources of these essential amino acids, one of which is methionine.

Methionine is vital for the healthy horse but is highly toxic in excess. A well-balanced diet containing adequate protein levels (10-12 per cent protein) will not be deficient in methionine.
The effect of excess methionine on the hoof horn is the progressive degeneration of the hoof horn, spreading outwards from the white line. The horse will be intermittently lame, with sore feet and have difficulty holding the shoe on for more than a few days.

Excess methionine can cause depletion of zinc, copper and iron and can lead to growth of weak, parakeratinized horn, typical of zinc deficiency. If the methionine supplement is omitted from the diet, the feet will recover.

Susan A. Kempson

Vitamin A

A recent fashion is the feeding of "feed balancers". Many of these are based on milk by-products and contain high levels of the fat-soluble vitamins, vitamin A and vitamin D. When fed with large quantities of carrots, horses show the detrimental effects of excess vitamin A. The results of excess vitamin A on the skin are well known.

Horses receiving toxic levels of vitamin A show a breakdown in the intertubular horn of the dorsal wall. This creates a fringe effect on the distal wall, the horn resembles spaghetti. The horn will also show exceptionally high levels of bacteria and fungi. At a cellular level, the intercellular lipids of the intertubular horn are altered and unable to fulfil their function. The different lipids of the tubular horn remain intact, creating the fringe effect. The dorsal wall takes a "glassy" appearance in these horses, before it breaks down completely at the distal border.

Excess carbohydrates

In dairy cattle, a diet containing excess carbohydrates has been shown to change the fatty acids in the cell membranes of the horn to trans-fatty acids. This weakens the cells, the intercellular lipids and makes the horn particularly susceptible to bacterial infection.

Similar problems are becoming manifest in horses. Many horse with while line disease have diets too high in carbohydrates. Treatment of the infection alone will not reduce the white line disease. Topical treatment alone will not solve the problem. A reduction in dietary carbohydrate and a change to a high fibre diet is required to accompany the topical antimicrobial therapy.

Laminitis

This is a subject worthy of a paper of its own. Much has been writeen about the aetiology and pathogenesis of laminitis. However, it is this author's belief that the majority of laminitis is due to changes and disruption of the gut microbial population. There are several different causes of changes in the equine gut flora which will lead to laminitis. One worth a mention, is the effect of clover. The cyanides in clover will

kill susceptible bacteria, creating an imbalance in the gut flora. This can lead to nutrient deficiencies as well as excess endotoxins.
A healthy gut flora in the horse is little understood, but is increasingly coming under threat from nutritional fads and fashions.

Nutritional management of hoof disease

Diet has a profound effect on the health of the hoof horn. Not only does it cause a breakdown in the structure but it also renders the horn susceptible to infection.

The diet and management of the horse must be examined carefully to excesses and imbalances. The author's recommendation for a horse with a grass/hay based diet is to provide feed of a hard alfalfa-based chaff and an energy source such as sugar beet pulp, oats, barley or a mix. Only one supplement should be fed at a time and the author recommends "Farrier's Formula" (Life Data Labs Inc, USA) as the best supplement to stimulate good quality hoof horn growth.

It is best to avoid silage or haylages for horses with poor quality hoof horn. The acidity and high protein levels of some haylages can lead to disruption of the gut flora which, in turn, causes deficiencies of some nutrients.

The micro-organisms must be reduced using a topical disinfectant (Life Data's Hoof Disinfectant) or antibiotic. Greasy hoof dressings or those containing fat solvents must be avoided at all times. Formaldehyde-based dressings will cross-link the proteins and render the horn brittle and more susceptible to cracks.

Horses suffering from laminitis will benefit from the addition of 500-1000 mg per day of magnesium oxide with vitamin B6. Tyrosine supplement at a rate of 300-500 mg per day will help horses with Cushing's disease and associated laminitis.

The secret of good nutrition is balance. Too many horses suffer from "a little does some good so a lot must do much more good". With horse, as well as human, nutrition, "keep it simple, keep it natural and keep it balanced" is a good maxim. The feet will benefit and the horse will thrive.

Susan A. Kempson

References

Kempson, S.A., 1987. A scanning electron microscopic study of hoof horn from horses with brittle feet. Vet. Record, 120, 586-587.

Kempson, S.A., 1990. Ultrastructural observations on the response on equine hoof defects to dietary supplementation - a scanning electron microscopic study. Vet. Record, 124, 37-40.

Kempson, S.A., and Campbell, E.H., 1998. The permeability barrier of the dorsal wall of the hoof capsule. Equine Veterinary Journal, Suppl.(26), 15-21.

Kempson, S.A. and Robb, R., 2004. Use of a topical disinfectant as part of a hoof care programme for horses with diseases of the hoof capsule. Vet. Record, 154, 647-652.

Anti-inflammatory and anti-oxidative feed ingredients

Pierre Lekeux and Brieuc de Moffarts
Department of physiology and sport medicine, Faculty of veterinary medicine, University of Liege, Belgium

Introduction

Recurrent inflammation and oxidative stress are frequent problems in sport horses, with negative effect on the health, the well-being and the performance of the animal. It is therefore necessary to develop curative and preventive strategies in order to control these problems.

Because of the huge costs requested for the development and registration of drugs specifically devoted to the equine species, ie a small market when compared to production animals and pet, the number of newly registered equine compounds have decreased dramatically. As a result more and more nutraceuticals are now proposed in order to prevent or modulate inflammation and/or oxidative stress in horses. A nutraceutical could be defined as a product intended to supplement the diet that contains at least one of the following substances: vitamin, mineral, herb or other botanical, amino acid, dietary substance for use to supplement the diet by increasing intake, and concentrate, metabolite, constituent, extract, or combination of any of the previously mentioned ingredients.

One of the problems for the clients is the frequent lack of scientific evidence concerning their quality, bioavailability, and in vitro and in vivo activity. Indeed scientific-based medicine is often lacking for most of the proposed products and replaced by theoretical and anecdotical considerations supported by a strong marketing. It is true that randomised, controlled, and blinded clinical trials are a difficult and expensive challenge in the equine practice. On the other hand, observational, descriptive, and anecdotal studies do not provide proof of efficacy.

Recent studies have demonstrated that some feed ingredients can be validated by scientific evidence, if a sufficient amount of money is devoted to it.

Major target: the persistent inflammatory reaction

Primarily the inflammatory cascade is beneficial for the cure of the patient by contributing to the destruction of the aggressors and the cicatrisation of the damaged tissues, eg by the release of free radicals and proteases and by many other mechanisms. Unfortunately the inflammatory reaction is sometimes excessive in intensity or duration. As a result, severe dysfunctions and lesions may occur and be responsible for poor performance or, in some cases, the development of irreversible damages. However a modulation of this deleterious inflammation is not easy, mainly because many cells and mediators (transcription factors, cytokines, chemokines, autacoids, neuropeptides, ..) are involved in this cascade where several pathways may act simultaneously, including endogenous antiinflammatory ones.

Because inflammation results mainly from an exaggerated expression of inflammatory genes, recent studies aimed at identifying the mechanisms implicated in this inappropriate inflammatory genes induction in horses. This is interesting since any pathway of the inflammatory cascade may be a potential target for nutraceuticals.

Main inflammatory genes encode (a) proinflammatory cytokines, including interleukin-1β (IL-1β) and tumor necrosis factor-α (TNF-α), which amplify pulmonary inflammation, (b) chemokines, such as interleukin-8 (IL-8), macrophage inflammatory protein-1α (MIP-1α), macrophage chemotactic protein-3 (MCP-3), RANTES (Regulated on Activation Normal T-cell Expressed and Secreted) and eotaxin, which are chemotactic for leukocytes, (c) adhesion factors, including intracellular adhesion molecule-1 (ICAM-1), vascular cell adhesion molecule-1 (VCAM-1) and E-selectin, which play a cardinal role in leukocyte recruitment, margination, diapedesis and transepithelial migration, and (d) inflammatory enzymes, such as cytosolic phospholipase A2 (cPLA2), inducible cyclooxygenase (COX-2) and inducible nitric oxide synthase (iNOS), which generate inflammatory mediators. All these inflammatory genes have been shown to contain κB sites for the transcription factor, nuclear factor κB (NF-κB), within their promoter or enhancer and therefore to depend on NF-κB for their expression, suggesting that this transcription factor could play a key role in the pathophysiology of equine airway inflammation.

NF-κB is highly activated in bronchial brushing samples (BBSs) and broncho-alveolar lavage (BAL) cells obtained from affected horses, as compared with healthy horses. Three weeks after antigen eviction, NF-κB activity in BBSs and BAL cells from diseased horses is generally maintained at moderate or high levels, and is highly correlated ($r = 0.88$) to the degree of residual lung dysfunction (Bureau *et al.*, 2000). Consequently, NF-κB could be a putative target in the therapy of persistent airway inflammation.

As a result, it was interesting to investigate if a selective blockade of NF-kappa B activity in airway immune cells inhibits the effector phase of experimental airway inflammation (Desmet *et al.*, 2004). We have assessed in an animal model of asthma the effects of selectively antagonizing NF-kappaB activity in the lungs. Intratracheal administration of NF-kappaB decoy oligodeoxynucleotides to asthmatic mice led to efficient nuclear transfection of airway immune cells, but not constitutive lung cells and draining lymph node cells, associated with abrogation of NF-kappaB activity in the airways upon allergic challenge. NF-kappaB inhibition was associated with strong attenuation of allergic lung inflammation, airway hyperresponsiveness, and local production of mucus. This study demonstrates for the first time that activation of NF-kappaB in local immune cells is critically involved in the effector phase of allergic airway disease and that specific NF-kappaB inhibition in the lungs has therapeutic potential in the control of pulmonary inflammation. Similar results have been obtained with another transcription factor, ie AP-1.

Since many genes, transcription factors and proteins are involved in the inflammatory cascade, a key question remains: which pathway needs to be inhibited or boosted in order to inhibit the deleterious effects of inflammation without significant side effects on the organism? In other words, it is crucial to identify which pro- or anti-inflammatory genes are over- or under-expressed in the local and inflammatory cells in the airways of horses with persistent inflammation. The current availability of the micro-array technology (see Thomas *et al.*, 2005, for a review) and the cloning of the equine genes involved in the inflammatory cascade could provide us with useful information in order to develop efficient strategies to modulate inappropriate inflammation, eg by inhibiting the over-expression of proinflammatory genes or by stimulating the expression of antiinflammatory genes. This promising approach is already under investigation in horses suffering from persistent inflammation.

Another target: the oxidative stress

For most animal species, oxygen is indispensable because it is the basal element of the body's energy production. However, a small percentage of inspired oxygen may not be used adequately and becomes "hyper-reactive". These forms of oxygen are called pro-oxidants.

On one hand, pro-oxidants have a beneficial effect by defending the organism against bacteriological or viral infections. On the other hand, an excessive generation of pro-oxidants might lead to cell damage. Such oxidative processes favour aging, as observed in fruits, vegetables and other biological products (putrefaction).

Against these pro-oxidants, the organism is naturally equipped with anti-oxidants such as enzymes, vitamins, trace elements and other molecules.

In horses in optimal physical condition, the oxidant and anti-oxidant balance is equilibrated.

Oxidative stress is defined as an imbalance between the endogenous antioxidant defence of the organism and the exogenous or endogenous pro-oxidant burden in favour of pro-oxidants. Pro-oxidants are highly reactive molecules able to induce cellular damage by oxidation of cellular components, such as lipids, proteins, nucleic acids and carbohydrates. These "reactive oxygen species" (ROS) are generated by three physiologic processes:

1. Leukocytes release important amounts of ROS during inflammation (respiratory burst).
2. Incomplete oxygen reduction by mitochondria leads to formation and release of ROS.
3. Several enzymes generate ROS as by-products of metabolic processes.

Antioxidants, such as vitamin A, C and E, glutathione, flavonoids, uric acid etc., are able to transform or inactivate ROS into less reactive molecules. Antioxidants are therefore essential to prevent cellular damage by pro-oxidants.

Antioxidant defences

The balance between positive and negative effects of ROS is thus particularly fragile. AOS production is strictly regulated by our organism, which has developed antioxidant defences that protect us against the potentially destructive effects of ROS. These defence systems consist of:
- enzymes (Cu-Zn and Mn superoxide dismutases, catalase, glutathione peroxidases, the thioredoxin/thioredoxin reductase pair, haem oxygenase, heat shock proteins);
- iron- and copper-transporting proteins (transferrin, ferritin, ceruleoplasmin);
- small antioxidant molecules (glutathione, uric acid, bilirubin, glucose, vitamins A, C, E, ubiquinone, carotenoids, flavonoids);
- oligoelements (copper, zinc, selenium) indispensable to the activity of antioxidant enzymes.

Alongside this panoply of defences against ROS is a secondary defence system consisting of enzymes whose role is to prevent intracellular accumulation of oxidised DNA or proteins and to degrade their toxic fragments.

Exercise induces oxidative stress

It has been demonstrated in scientific studies (Mills *et al.*, 1996; Kirschvink *et al.*, 1999; de Moffarts *et al.*, 2004a) that intense exercise induces oxidative stress in horses.

When oxygen consumption increases, oxidative processes are gaining importance. The horse is an exceptional athlete able to increase 30 times its oxygen consumption. Given that 2 to 5 % of inspired oxygen is converted within the cells into pro-oxidants, the exercising horse is particularly exposed to oxidative processes.

Pierre Lekeux and Brieuc de Moffarts

Overtraining and competition periods induce oxidative stress

This work illustrates that intensively trained horses undergo, since the beginning of the racing period a decrease of their anti-oxidant defence (de Moffarts *et al.*, 2004b).

Effect of oxidative stress on the health of the horse

Intensive exercise leads to an increase of the pro-oxidative burden, which might generate an oxidative stress (a disequilibrium between the anti-oxidant defence of the organism and the pro-oxidant burden) and which might favour the development of pathologies.

Exercise-induced oxidative stress might lead to exercise intolerance or poor performance. As oxidative processes are implied in development of disease and especially in development of muscle lesions, poor performance might be a consequence of oxidative stress.

Correlation studies between performance parameters of sport horses and antioxidants have been performed (unpublished data). These studies have shown that horses with best performances are those with an optimal and equilibrated oxidant status.

In this study including 45 horses, the horses being considered as the best competitors by their trainer were those with the highest lipophilic antioxidant capacity of plasma and the lowest lipid peroxidation.

It has been shown that oxidative stress might favour the development of problems associated with:
■ the locomotor system (myopathies, arthrosis, ...) (Auer *et al.*, 1993; Perkins *et al.*, 1998);
■ the respiratory system (tracheobronchitis, small airway inflammation) (Art *et al.*, 1999; Kirschvink *et al.*, 2001);
■ the vascular system (exercise-induced pulmonary haemorrhage) (Derksen, 1997);
■ the nervous system (motor neuron disease, grass sickness) (Divers *et al.*, 1994; Polack *et al.*, 2000).

Table 1. Major markers of oxidative stress which can be accurately measured in horses.

Markers	Type	Role	Observation
Ascorbic acid (AA or VitC)	Hydrophilic antioxidant	Mostly plasmatic element. The first barrier against pro-oxidant.	It is the most sensitive (AA or Vit C) vitamin.
Glutathione reduced forms (GSH)	Hydrophilic antioxidant	Mostly cytoplasmic element protecting the protein against pro-oxidant	Depletion during exercise and disease.
Glutathione oxidised forms (GSSG)	Oxidant marker	Oxidised forms of GSH are sensitive markers of oxidative process	Increased during exercise and disease
Antioxidant capacity of water soluble components in plasma (ACW)	Antioxidant marker	Marker of the capacity of the plasma to react against the pro-oxidant (hydrophilic part)	Correlated with AA
Antioxidant capacity of lipid soluble components in plasma (ACL)	Antioxidant marker	Marker of the capacity of the plasma to react against the pro-oxidant (lipophilic part).	Correlated with Vit E and β-car
α-tocopherol (Vit E)	Lipophilic antioxidant	Vitamin protecting the lipid against pro-oxidants	Decreased during repetitive exercise.
β-carotene (β-car)	Lipophilic antioxidant	Pro-vitamin A and element for protection against singlet oxygen pro-oxidant.	
Selenium (Se)	Trace-element	Catalytic element for GPx effectiveness.	Se and Vit E deficiency is associated with myopathy.
Copper (Cu)	Trace-element	Catalytic element for SOD effectiveness.	
Zinc (Zn)	Trace-element	Catalytic element for SOD effectiveness.	
Superoxide dismutase (SOD)	Enzymatic antioxidant	Antioxidant enzyme protecting against superoxide anion (pro-oxidant).	Improved with training and decreased during oxidative process
Glutathione peroxidase (GPx)	Enzymatic antioxidant	Antioxidant enzyme regenerating glutathione.	Correlated with Se. Improved with training and decreased during overexercising
Lipid Peroxide (Pool)	Oxidant marker	Follows the lipid oxidative processes.	Negatively correlated with Vit E. Low in the good horses.
Oxidised Protein (Protox)	Oxidant marker	Follows the proteic oxidative processes.	Increase with exercise and pathology

Markers of oxidative stress

The markers of the oxidative stress have been validated for the equine species (Kirschvink *et al.*, de Moffarts *et al.*, Deaton *et al*). The most frequently used ones are listed in table 1.

Modulation of inflammation and oxidative stress in horses

By training

It has been shown in a study (de Moffarts *et al.*, 2004a) that appropriate training allows to increase the antioxidant defence in horses (thereby increasing its resistance against pro-oxidants and reducing the oxidative stress-related inflammatory disorders).

By feed ingredients/nutraceuticals

Several studies have shown that oxidative stress and/or inflammation in horses receiving an adapted cocktail might be prevented and/or counterbalanced. The published scientific studies are listed in the section Further readings. Some of them are briefly described here.

Examples of scientific studies on feed ingredients in horses

Bioavailability

Evidence of the oral absorption of chondroitin sulfate has been shown in the horse. The oral bioavailability of 8.0-kDa chondroitin sulfate was 32% compared with 22% for 16.9-kDa chondroitin sulfate. The oral bioavailability of glucosamine hydrochloride in horses was found to be 2.5% with a large volume of distribution, which the clinicians interpreted as poor absorption from the intestinal tract and extensive tissue uptake (Eddington *et al.*, 2001). A more recent publication confirmed that after oral dosing, the mean C_{max} for glucosamine was 10.6 µg/ml, and the mean bioavailability was 2.5%. This was interpreted as providing evidence that glucosamine is absorbed orally, albeit it low, and that it is most likely due to extensive first pass metabolism in the gastrointestinal tract and/or liver before systemic availability (Adebowale *et al.*, 2002).

In vitro studies

For instance, these studies help to determine at what concentration the feed additives might have an effect. In a study with articular cartilage obtained from antebrachiocarpal and middle carpal joints of horses, explant discs were treated with lipopolysaccharide or recombinant human interleukin-1 to induce cartilage degradation. Three concentrations of glucosamine (0.25, 2.5, or 25 mg/ml) were tested. The results showed that maximal NO production, proteoglycan release, and MMP activity were detected 1 day after the addition of LPS or recombinant IL-1β to the media. The addition of 25 mg/ml glucosamine prevented the increase in NO production, proteoglycan release, and MMP activity induced by LPS, or rhIL-1 (Fenton *et al.*, 2000).

Ex vivo studies

The effect of an oral supplementation on erythrocyte membrane fluidity was investigated in exercising horses. Twelve healthy and regularly trained horses were randomly divided in two groups; group 1 received during 4 weeks an oral antioxidant cocktail enriched with (n-3 fatty acids, whereas group 2 was placebo-treated. At the end of the treatment period, all horses performed a standardized exercise test (SET) under field conditions. Venous blood was sampled before starting the treatment (T0), immediately before (R) as well as 15 min (E15') and 24 hours (E24h) after the SET. Assessment of the erythrocyte membrane fluidity (EMS) was determined by electron spin resonance using the relaxation-contraction time (the relaxation contraxion time (Tc) being inversely proportional to EMF).

The SET induced a significant ($p < 0.05$) increase of Tc. Tc significantly increased in placebo-treated horses (R versus E15'), which was not the case for horses receiving the feed supplement (de Moffarts *et al.*, 2004).

In vivo studies in experimental conditions

An oxidant/antioxidant imbalance in favour of oxidants has been identified as playing a decisive role in the pathogenesis of chronic inflammatory airway diseases. Nutritional antioxidant supplementation might reduce oxidative damage by enhancement of the antioxidant defence, thereby modulating inflammatory processes. In a placebo-controlled, blind study, it was tested whether a dietary antioxidant supplement administered for 4 weeks would improve lung function and reduce airway inflammation in heaves-affected horses. Eight horses in clinical remission of heaves were investigated at rest and after a standardised exercise test before and after treatment with an antioxidant supplement (consisting of a mixture of natural antioxidants including vitamins E and C and selenium from a variety of sources) or placebo (oatfeed pellets without additive). Pulmonary function and exercise tolerance were monitored; systemic and pulmonary lining fluid uric acid, glutathione and 8-epi-PGF(2alpha) were analysed, and bronchoalveolar lavage (BAL) cytology and inflammatory scoring of the airways were performed. The antioxidant treatment significantly improved exercise tolerance and significantly reduced endoscopic inflammatory score. Plasma uric acid concentrations were significantly reduced, suggesting downregulation of the xanthine-dehydrogenase and xanthine-oxydase pathway. Haemolysate glutathione showed a nonsignificant trend to increase, while plasma 8-epi-PGF(2alpha) remained unchanged. Pulmonary markers and BAL cytology were not significantly affected by antioxidant supplementation. The present study suggests that the antioxidant supplement tested modulated oxidant/antioxidant balance and airway inflammation of heaves-affected horses (Kirschvink *et al.*, 2002).

Another study was to quantify the effect of flaxseed *(Linum usitatissimum)* supplementation on the skin test response of atopic horses. Six horses that displayed a positive skin test for allergy to extract from *Culicoides* sp. participated in the 42-day, placebo-controlled, double-blind, cross-over trial. Results showed that supplementation with flaxseed for 42 days in our experimental horses reduced the mean skin test response to *Culicoides* sp. This observation was concurrent with a significant decrease in the long-chain saturated fatty acids; behenic acid (22:0) and lignoceric acid (24:0), in the hair of horses receiving flaxseed. There was also a significant decrease in aspartate aminotransferase, and increase in serum glucose in the treatment animals at specific sampling points. It was concluded that; in this small pilot study, flaxseed was able to reduce the lesional area of the skin test response of atopic horses, alter the fatty acid profile of the hair, reduce inflammation, and did not elicit any negative side-effects in the experimental horses (O'Neill *et al.*, 2002).

In vivo studies in field conditions

The effect of oral antioxidant complementation has been tested on blood oxidant markers in trained Thoroughbred horses. The oxidant/antioxidant equilibrium was assessed at three occasions during a period of three months under field conditions by blood oxidant markers analysis, *i.e.* ascorbic acid (AA), antioxidant capacity of water soluble components (ACW), reduced (GSH) and oxidised (GSSG) glutathione, α-tocopherol, β-carotene, antioxidant capacity of lipid soluble components (ACL), superoxide dismutase (SOD), glutathione-peroxidase (GPx) and trace-elements, *i.e.* selenium (Se), copper (Cu), zinc (Zn). Two groups of horses were randomly formed; ten horses received a placebo, 30 horses were orally supplemented by an antioxidant mixture. An oxidant/antioxidant imbalance was observed during the three-months period in the placebo-treated group and was mainly reflected by a decrease of GSH, SOD, GPx and Se as well as an increase of GSSG. The antioxidant supplement prevented GPx and Se decrease and increased ACW, α-tocopherol, β-carotene and ACL. Supplement-treated horses also showed significantly lower creatine phosphokinase (CPK) values than placebo-treated horses. At T0, significant sex- or age-related differences were found for AA, ACW, α-tocopherol, SOD; GPx and Se. Regression analyses between markers revealed significant correlations for the following markers: ACW-AA, ACL-α-tocopherol, GPx-Se, CPK-Se, CPK-α-tocopherol and CPK-Cu. This field study has shown that trained thoroughbred horses undergo significant changes of their blood oxidant/antioxidant balance and that oral antioxidant supplementation might partially counterbalance these changes by improving the hydrophilic, lipophilic and enzymatic antioxidant blood capacity (de Moffarts *et al.*, 2005).

In another study, the effect of dietary fish oil supplementation was tested on exercising horses. Ten horses of Thoroughbred or Standardbred breeding were used to study the effects of dietary fish oil supplementation on the metabolic response to a high-intensity incremental exercise test. Horses were assigned to either a fish oil (n = 6) or corn oil (n = 4) treatment. During exercise, horses receiving fish oil had a lower heart rate (treatment × time interaction; $P < 0.05$)

and tended to have lower packed cell volume (treatment effect; $P = 0.087$). Plasma lactate concentrations were not affected by treatment. Plasma glucose concentrations were not different between groups during exercise but were lower (treatment × time interaction; $P < 0.01$) for the fish oil group during recovery. Serum insulin tended to be lower in fish oil horses throughout exercise (treatment effect; $P = 0.064$). There was a tendency for glucose : insulin ratios to be higher for fish oil-treated horses throughout exercise (treatment effect; $P = 0.065$). Plasma FFA were lower (treatment × time interaction; $P < 0.01$) in horses receiving fish oil than in horses receiving corn oil during the initial stages of the exercise test. Serum glycerol concentrations also were lower in fish oil-treated horses $(P < 0.05)$. Serum cholesterol concentrations were lower in horses receiving fish oil (treatment effect; $P < 0.05$), but serum triglycerides were not affected by treatment $(P = 0.55)$. These data suggest that addition of fish oil to the diet alters exercise metabolism in conditioned horses (O'Connor *et al.*, 2004).

References

Adebowale A, Du J, Liang Z, *et al.* 2002. The bioavailability and pharmacokinetics of glucosamine hydrochloride and low molecular weight chondroitin sulfate after single and multiple doses to beagle dogs. Biopharm Drug Dispos; 23:217-225.

Art T, Kirschvink N, Smith N, Votion D, Lekeux P. 1999. Cardiorespiratory measurements and indices of oxidative stress in exercising COPD horses. Equine Vet J Suppl. Jul;30:83-7.

Art T, Kirschvink N, Smith N, Lekeux P. 1999. Indices of oxidative stress in blood and pulmonary epithelium lining fluid in horses suffering from recurrent airway obstruction. Equine Vet J. Sep;31(5):397-401.

Bureau F, Bonizzi G, Kirschvink N, Desmecht D, Merville MP, Bours V, Lekeux P. 2000. Correlation between nuclear factor-kappaB activity in bronchial brushing samples and lung dysfunction in an animal model of asthma. Am J Respir Crit Care Med. Apr;161(4 Pt 1):1314-21.

Deaton CM, Marlin DJ, Roberts CA, Smith N, Harris PA, Kelly FJ, Schroter RC., 2002. Antioxidant supplementation and pulmonary function at rest and exercise. Equine Vet J Suppl. Sep;(34):58-65.

de Moffarts B., Portier K., Kirschvink N., Pincemail J., Lekeux P., 2004. Effect of exercise and oral antioxidant supplementation on blood oxidant markers and erythrocyte membrane fluidity in horses. Free Radical Biology and Medicine volume 37, Suppl 1, S33 de Moffarts B, Kirschvink N, Art T, Pincemail J, Lekeux P. 2005. Effect of oral antioxidant supplementation on blood antioxidant status in trained thoroughbred horses. Vet J. Jan;169(1):65-74.

Eddington ND, Du J, White N. 2001. Evidence of the oral absorption of chondroitin sulfate as determined by total disaccharide content after oral and intravenous administration to horses. In: Proceedings of the 47th Ann Am Assoc Equine Practitioners Convention 2001; 326-328.

Kirschvink N, Fievez L, Bougnet V, Art T, Degand G, Smith N, Marlin D, Roberts C, Harris P, Lekeux P. Effect of nutritional antioxidant supplementation on systemic and pulmonary antioxidant status, airway inflammation and lung function in heaves-affected horses.

Fenton JI, Chlebek-Brown KA, Peters TL, *et al*. 2002. Glucosamine HCl reduces equine articular degradation in explant cultures. Osteoarthritis Cartilage 2000; 6:258-265. Equine Vet J. Nov;34(7):705-12.

Kirschvink N, Art T, de Moffarts B, Smith N, Marlin D, Roberts C, Lekeux P., 2002. Relationship between markers of blood oxidant status and physiological variables in healthy and heaves-affected horses after exercise. Equine Vet J Suppl. Sep;(34):159-64.

Kirschvink N, Smith N, Fievez L, Bougnet V, Art T, Degand G, Marlin D, Roberts C, Genicot B, Lindsey P, Lekeux P. Effect of chronic airway inflammation and exercise on pulmonary and systemic antioxidant status of healthy and heaves-affected horses. Equine Vet J. 2002 Sep;34(6):563-71.

Marlin DJ, Johnson L, Kingston DA, Smith NC, Deaton CM, Mann S, Heaton P, Van Vugt F, Saunders K, Kydd J, Harris PA., 2004. Application of the comet assay for investigation of oxidative DNA damage in equine peripheral blood mononuclear cells. J Nutr. Aug;134(8 Suppl):2133S-2140S.

Marlin DJ, Fenn K, Smith N, Deaton CD, Roberts CA, Harris PA, Dunster C, Kelly FJ., 2002. Changes in circulatory antioxidant status in horses during prolonged exercise. J Nutr. Jun;132(6 Suppl 2):1622S-7S.

Mills PC, Smith NC, Casas I, Harris P, Harris RC, Marlin DJ., 1996. Effects of exercise intensity and environmental stress on indices of oxidative stress and iron homeostasis during exercise in the horse. Eur J Appl Physiol Occup Physiol.;74(1-2):60-6.

O'Connor CI, Lawrence LM, Lawrence AC, Janicki KM, Warren LK, Hayes S., 2004. The effect of dietary fish oil supplementation on exercising horses. J Anim Sci. Oct;82(10):2978-84.

O'Neill W, McKee S, Clarke AF., 2002. Flaxseed (Linum usitatissimum) supplementation associated with reduced skin test lesional area in horses with Culicoides hypersensitivity. Can J Vet Res. Oct;66(4):272-7.

www

McIlwraiht CW. Licensed Medications, "Generic" Medications, Compounding, and Nutraceuticals - What Has Been Scientifically Validated, where Do We Encounter Scientific Mistruth, and where Are We Legally? Internet Publisher: International Veterinary Information Service, Ithaca NY (www.ivis.org), 4-Dec-2004; P1482.1204.

Probiox website: http://www.probiox.com/uk/index_uk.htm

An extensive review on markers of the oxidative stress in veterinary medicine can be found at http://www.probiox.com

Nutrition of the growing horse: Feeding management to reduce DOD

Joe D. Pagan
Kentucky Equine Research, Versailles, Kentucky, USA

Introduction

Nutrition may play an important role in the pathogenesis of developmental orthopedic disease in horses. Deficiencies, excesses, and imbalances of nutrients may result in an increase in both the incidence and severity of physitis, angular limb deformity, wobbler syndrome (wobbles), and osteochondritis dissecans (OCD).

Nutritional factors as a cause of developmental orthopedic disease

Mineral deficiencies

A deficiency of minerals, including calcium, phosphorus, copper and zinc, may lead to developmental orthopedic disease. The ration of a growing horse should be properly fortified because most commonly fed cereal grains and forages contain insufficient quantities of several minerals. A ration of grass hay and oats would only supply about 40% and 70% of a weanling's calcium and phosphorus requirement, respectively, and less than 40% of its requirement for copper and zinc (Table 1). The best method of diagnosing mineral deficiencies is through ration evaluation. Blood, hair, and hoof analysis is of limited usefulness.

Mineral excesses

Horses can tolerate fairly high levels of mineral intake, but excesses of calcium, phosphorus, zinc, iodine, fluoride, and certain heavy metals such as lead and cadmium, may lead to developmental orthopedic disease (Table 2).

Joe D. Pagan

Table 1. Mineral requirements for weanlings.

Nutrient concentration required in total diet (90% dry basis)		Grass hay	Alfalfa hay	Oats	Corn	Barley
Moderate growth	Rapid growth					
Calcium (%) .62	.70	.35	1.25	.08	.05	.05
Phosphorus (%) .40	.45	.20	.22	.34	.27	.34
Zinc (ppm) 65	65	9	16	6	4	8
Copper (ppm) 22	22	17	28	35	19	17

Table 2. Toxic mineral levels (adapted from Cunha, 1997 and NRC, 1989).

Mineral	Level of mineral needed by young horse (ppm)	Level at which mineral is toxic (ppm)
Zinc	60-70	9000
Iodine	0.2-0.3	5.0
Fluoride	–	50
Lead	–	80
Selenium	0.2-0.3	5.0
Manganese	60-70	4000
Copper	20-30	300-500
Cobalt	0.1	400
Iron	125	5000

Mineral excesses occur because of overfortification or environmental contamination. Massive oversupplementation of calcium (>300% of required) may lead to a secondary mineral deficiency by interfering with the absorption of other minerals such as phosphorus, zinc, and iodine. Excessive calcium intake may be compounded by the use of legume hays as the primary forage source. Iodine and selenium oversupplementation occurs if supplements are fed at inappropriate levels. A ration evaluation is the best way to identify this type of mineral imbalance.

Environmental contamination is a more likely cause of developmental orthopedic disease because contamination may result in extremely high intakes of potentially toxic minerals. If a farm is experiencing an unusually high incidence of developmental orthopedic disease or if the location and severity of skeletal lesions are abnormal, environmental contamination should be investigated. Blood, feed, and water analysis should be performed. In addition, chemical analysis of hoof and hair samples may reveal valuable information in such a situation. Farms that are located near factories or smelters are the most likely candidates for this type of contamination, although OCD from a zinc-induced copper deficiency has been reported on farms using fence paint containing zinc or galvanized water pipes.

Mineral imbalances

The ratio of minerals may be as important as the actual amount of individual minerals in the ration. High levels of phosphorus in the ration will inhibit the absorption of calcium and will lead to a deficiency, even if the amount of calcium present was normally adequate. The ratio of calcium to phosphorus in the ration of young horses should never dip below 1:1 and ideally it should be 1.5:1. Too much calcium may affect phosphorus status, particularly if the level of phosphorus in the ration is marginal. Calcium to phosphorus ratios greater than 2.5:1 should be avoided if possible. Forage diets with high calcium levels should be supplemented with phosphorus. The ratio of zinc to copper should be 3:1 to 4:1.

Dietary energy excess

Excessive energy intake can lead to rapid growth and increased body fat, which may predispose young horses to developmental orthopedic disease. A recent Kentucky study showed that growth rate and body size may increase the incidence of certain types of developmental orthopedic disease in Thoroughbred foals (Pagan *et al.*, 1996). Yearlings that showed osteochondrosis of the hock and stifle were large at birth, grew rapidly from 3 to 8 months of age, and were heavier than the average population as weanlings.

The source of calories for young horses may also be important, as hyperglycemia or hyperinsulinemia have been implicated in the pathogenesis of osteochondrosis (Glade *et al.*, 1984; Ralston, 1995). Foals that experience an exaggerated and sustained increase in circulating glucose or insulin in response to a carbohydrate (grain) meal may be predisposed to development of osteochondrosis. In vitro studies with fetal and foal chondrocytes suggest that the role of insulin in growth cartilage may be to promote chondrocyte survival or to suppress differentiation and that hyperinsulinemia may be a contributory factor to equine osteochondrosis (Henson *et al.*, 1997).

Recent research from Kentucky Equine Research (Pagan *et al.*, 2001) suggests that hyperinsulinemia may influence the incidence of OCD in Thoroughbred weanlings. In a large field trial, 218 Thoroughbred weanlings (average age 300 ± 40 days, average body weight 300 kg ± 43 kg) were studied. A glycemic response test was conducted by feeding a meal that consisted of the weanling's normal concentrate at a level of intake equal to 1.4 g nonstructural carbohydrate (NSC) per kilogram body weight. A single blood sample was taken 120 minutes post feeding for the determination of glucose and insulin.

In this study, a high glucose and insulin response to a concentrate meal was associated with an increased incidence of OCD. Glycemic responses measured in the weanlings were highly correlated with each feed's glycemic index (GI), suggesting that the GI of a farm's feed may play a role in the pathogenesis of OCD. Glycemic index characterizes the rate of carbohydrate absorption after a meal and is defined as the area under the glucose response curve after consumption of a measured amount of carbohydrate from a test feed divided by the area under the curve after consumption of a reference meal (Jenkins *et al.*, 1981). In rats, prolonged feeding of high GI feed results in basal hyperinsulinemia and an elevated insulin response to an intravenous glucose tolerance test (Pawlak *et al.*, 2001). Hyperinsulinemia may affect chondrocyte maturation, leading to altered matrix metabolism and faulty mineralization or altered cartilage growth by influencing other hormones such as thyroxine (Pagan *et al.*, 1996; Jeffcott and Henson, 1998).

Based on the results of this study, it would be prudent to feed foals concentrates that produce low glycemic responses. More research is needed to determine if the incidence of OCD can be reduced through this type of dietary management.

Feeding practices that contribute to developmental orthopedic disease

Several feeding scenarios may contribute to developmental orthopedic disease. Once identified, most can be easily corrected through adjustments in feed type and intake. Several of the most common mistakes made in feeding young growing horses are explained.

Overfeeding

One of the most common problems of feeding young horses is excessive intake that results in accelerated growth rate or fattening. Both conditions may contribute to developmental orthopedic disease. Unfortunately, there are no simple rules about how much grain is too much, because total intake of both forage and grain determines caloric consumption. Large intakes of grain are appropriate if the forage is sparse or poor quality, as often is the case in tropical environments. For example, grain intakes as high as 2% to 2.5% of body weight may be necessary to sustain reasonable growth in weanlings that have access to no forage other than tropic pasture. Conversely, grain intakes higher than 1% body weight may be considered excessive when weanlings are raised on lush temperate pasture or have access to high-quality alfalfa hay.

The surest way to document excessive intake is by weighing and using condition scoring in the growing horse. Growth rates and condition scores for Thoroughbred foals can be compared to the data presented in Table 3. Based on a system developed by Henneke *et al.* (1981), condition scoring measures fat deposition. Horses are scored from 1 to 9 with 1 denoting extreme thinness and 9 indicating obesity. In a Kentucky study, fillies tended to have higher condition scores than colts, and the difference was greatest at 4 months of age (fillies 6.48; colts 6.0). These condition scores are considered moderate to fleshy according to the Henneke scoring system. By 12 months of age, the condition scores of the colts and fillies had dropped to 5.3 and 5.4, respectively. Both sexes increased condition score slightly from 14 to 18 months.

If growth rate cannot be measured, excessive intake can often be assessed by ration evaluation. For example, a six-month-old

Table 3. Growth rates of fillies and colts in central Kentucky.

Average days of age	Colts BW (kg)	Fillies BW (kg)	Colts ADG (kg/d)	Fillies ADG (kg/d)	Colts HT* (cm)	Fillies HT* (cm)	Colts BCS**	Fillies BCS**
14	77.7	76.1	—	—	107.3	106.3	5.7	6.0
43	116.3	115.1	1.38	1.34	115.7	115.5	6.2	6.4
72	149.5	148.5	1.20	1.19	122.6	121.8	6.2	6.3
99	182.1	178.6	1.14	1.11	127.3	127.1	6.0	6.5
127	208.8	207.9	1.01	1.01	129.8	130.3	5.8	5.9
155	233.6	230.2	0.89	0.84	133.5	132.5	5.5	5.7
183	255.9	250.7	0.80	0.75	135.8	134.7	5.4	5.6
212	277.1	271.0	0.75	0.71	138.2	137.4	5.5	5.5
240	295.1	287.3	0.68	0.60	140.0	139.4	5.4	5.5
267	309.1	300.6	0.55	0.48	141.8	140.7	5.4	5.4
296	322.0	311.0	0.43	0.40	144.2	142.5	5.3	5.4
323	335.1	322.5	0.40	0.35	145.4	144.0	5.4	5.4
350	349.2	335.2	0.43	0.39	147.0	145.5	5.3	5.4
378	362.5	350.1	0.45	0.51	148.3	146.7	5.4	5.5
406	378.9	367.9	0.52	0.60	150.2	148.2	5.5	5.7
435	396.2	388.9	0.62	0.65	150.8	149.6	5.5	5.8
462	414.2	407.9	0.59	0.60	152.5	151.5	5.6	5.8
490	427.8	418.0	0.55	0.54	153.4	151.8	5.7	5.8

ADG = Average daily gain
*Height
**Body condition score

Thoroughbred weanling (250 kg body weight, 500 kg mature body weight) was being fed 4 kg/day of a 16% protein sweet feed and 2 kg of alfalfa hay and had access to high-quality fall Kentucky pasture. To support a reasonable rate of growth (0.80 kg/d), this weanling required about 17 Mcal of digestible energy per day. The hay and grain intake of this foal alone would supply about 17.5 Mcal of digestible energy, which is slightly above the weanling's requirement. If a reasonable level of pasture intake is included (1% of body weight or 2.5 kg dry matter), this weanling would be consuming 135% of its digestible energy requirement, a level likely to cause problems.

To reduce intake, the alfalfa hay should be eliminated, if the pasture is indeed adequate. If hay were needed when the weanling is stalled, grass hay would be more appropriate. Secondly, grain intake should be reduced to a level of about 3 kg/d. At this level of grain intake, the weanling would need to consume about 3.3 kg of pasture dry matter to support a growth rate of 0.80 kg/d, and the ration would be nicely balanced.

Inappropriate grain for forage being fed

Occasionally, the concentrate offered to a growing horse is incorrectly fortified to complement the forage that is being fed. The problem occurs particularly when the forage is mostly alfalfa or clover. Most concentrates for young horses are formulated with levels of minerals and protein needed to balance grass forage.

For example, a 12-month-old yearling (315 kg body weight, 500 kg mature body weight, 0.50 kg/d ADG) is raised without access to pasture and the only forage available is alfalfa hay, which is fed at a level of intake equal to 1.5% of the yearling's body weight (4.72 kg/d). At this level of forage intake, the yearling would only require about 2.5 kg of grain per day. If a typical 14% protein sweet feed that was formulated to balance grass forage is used, the ration would be inappropriate for a number of reasons. Calcium would be 183% of the yearling's requirement, with a calcium to phosphorus ratio of 2.9:1. This would not be a problem except that phosphorus and zinc are marginal in the ration. Because calcium may interfere with the absorption of both of these minerals, the yearling may be at risk of developmental orthopedic disease from a zinc or phosphorus deficiency. The solution is to feed a concentrate that is more appropriately balanced for legume hay. For example, a 12% protein feed with 0.4% calcium, 0.9% phosphorus, and 180 ppm zinc would be more suitable.

Inadequate fortification in grain

The most common reasons for inadequate fortification are using unfortified or underfortified grain mixes, using correctly fortified feeds at levels of intake that are below the manufacturer's recommendation, or using fortified feeds diluted with straight cereal grains. These errors in feeding can be corrected by the incorporation of a highly fortified grain balancer supplement.

Joe D. Pagan

For example, a 6-month-old weanling (200 kg body weight, 400 kg mature body weight, 0.60 kg/d ADG) is fed 3 kg/d of a 10% protein sweet feed that is intended for adult horses. To compound matters, the weanling is also fed grass hay with an estimated intake of 2.3 kg/d. This ration is deficient in protein, calcium, phosphorus, zinc, and copper. This foal would be prone to a rough hair coat and physitis. There are two ways to correct this problem. A properly formulated 14% to 16% protein grain mix with adequate mineral fortification could be used, or 1 kg of a grain balancer pellet can be substituted for 1 kg of the 10% sweet feed. This type of supplement is typically fortified with 25% to 30% protein, 2.5% to 3.0% calcium, 1.75% to 2.0% phosphorus, 125 to 175 ppm copper, and 375 to 475 ppm zinc. This is an extremely useful type of supplement to correct underfortified rations.

Feeding systems to prevent developmental orthopedic disease

Sucklings

If the broodmare has been fed properly during late pregnancy, it is unnecessary to supplement the suckling with minerals until it reaches 90 days of age. At 90 days, moderate amounts of a well-fortified foal feed can be introduced and gradually increased until the suckling is consuming around 0.5 kg feed per month of age. It is critical that the suckling be accustomed to eating grain before it is weaned. If it is not, there is a very good chance that there will be a dramatic decrease in growth rate at weaning. When the weanling finally starts eating grain, a compensatory growth spurt will occur that may result in developmental orthopedic disease.

Weanlings

The most critical stage of growth for preventing developmental orthopedic disease is from weaning to 12 months of age, when the skeleton is most vulnerable to disease and nutrient intake and balance is most important. Weanlings should be grown at a moderate rate with adequate mineral supplementation. In temperate regions, the contribution of pasture is often underestimated, leading to excessive growth rates and developmental orthopedic disease.

Yearlings

Once a horse reaches 12 months of age, it is much less likely to develop several forms of developmental orthopedic disease than a younger horse. Many of the lesions that become clinically relevant after this age are typically formed at a younger age. Still, proper nutrient balance remains important for the yearling. It is best to delay the increased energy intakes that are required for sales prepping as long as possible because the skeleton is less vulnerable to developmental orthopedic disease as the yearling ages. Normally, increasing energy intake 90 days before a sale is enough time to add the extra body condition that is often expected in a sales yearling.

Physitis in the carpus is often a major concern with sales yearlings. To reduce the incidence of physitis in these horses, the level of trace mineral supplementation should remain high and a significant portion of the energy normally supplied from grain should be replaced with fat and fermentable fiber. Sales preparation grain mixes can contain as much as 10% fat. Sources of fermentable fiber include beet pulp and soy hulls.

Nutritional management of developmental orthopedic disease

The goal of a feeding program for young horses is to reduce or eliminate the incidence of developmental orthopedic disease. Unfortunately, developmental orthopedic disease will still occur in some foals. Nutritional intervention can help reduce the severity of many forms of developmental orthopedic disease, but not all of the damage resulting from developmental orthopedic disease is reversible. However, it is important to alter the feeding programs of foals with developmental orthopedic disease. The type of alteration will follow a similar pattern but will depend on the foal's age and the type of developmental orthopedic disease. In almost every instance, energy intake should be reduced while maintaining adequate levels of protein and minerals. The rationale for this type of modification is that skeletal growth should be slowed, but adequate substrate should be available to promote healthy bone development.

Physitis

Grain intake should be restricted to a level supplying around 75% of the foal's normal energy requirement. This restriction, however, should not compromise protein and mineral intake, so a different type of feed formulation may be required. For instance, a six-month-old weanling (250 kg body weight, 500 kg mature body weight, 0.8 kg average daily growth) on a decent fall pasture would normally consume around 3.5 kg of a 16% protein foal feed. If this foal developed physitis, it would be confined and fed grass hay (3 kg/d). Reducing the grain intake to a level that was 75% of the foal's normal digestible energy would result in shortages of protein, lysine, calcium, and phosphorus. These shortfalls could be overcome by replacing 1 kg of the 16% percent sweet feed with a grain balancer pellet. This ration would supply 90% of the foal's normal protein requirement alone with a good supply of minerals. As the physitis resolves, intake of the 16% grain mix can be slowly increased and the supplement pellet intake slowly decreased until the foal returns to its normal ration.

Wobbler syndrome

A feeding program like the one described previously is also appropriate for the horse with wobbler syndrome except that the degree of exercise and energy restriction may be more severe. In this case, a feeding program that combined grass hay (2 kg/d) with a moderate amount of alfalfa hay (2 kg/d) and 1 kg/d of balancer pellet would result in a reduction in energy intake equal to 65% of normal intake while maintaining adequate levels of protein and mineral intake.

Osteochondritis dissecans

Once a foal develops osteochondritis dissecans that is severe enough to produce clinical signs, the effect of diet is going to be minimal in solving the existing lesion. Again, reducing energy intake and body weight while maintaining adequate protein and mineral intake is advised. Conservative management of shoulder (humeral head) and stifle (lateral trochlear ridge) OCD lesions has been successful. Complete stall rest is recommended along with intra-articular hyaluronan and intramuscular Adequan. There have been anecdotal reports of improvement in lesions identified radiographically through the use of oral joint supplements containing glucosamine and chondroitin sulfate, but these findings have not been validated in a controlled study.

Summary

Nutrition may play a role in the pathogenesis of developmental orthopedic disease. Mineral deficiencies, excesses, or imbalances may be involved along with excesses in energy or carbohydrate intake. A computerized ration evaluation is the best method to identify potential problems. The feeding errors that most often cause developmental orthopedic disease are excessive grain intake, an inappropriate grain mix for the forage being fed, and inadequate fortification in the grain. Each of these can easily be corrected by selecting an appropriate grain mix and feeding it at the correct level of intake. Foals that already have developmental orthopedic disease should have their energy intakes reduced while maintaining adequate levels of protein and mineral intake.

References

Cunha, T.J. 1997. Horse Feeding and Nutrition (2nd Ed.). Academic Press, Orlando, Florida.

Glade, M.J., S. Gupta, and T.J. Reimers. 1984. Hormonal responses to high and low planes of nutrition in weanling thoroughbreds. J. Anim. Sci. 59(3):658-665.

Henneke, D.R., G.D. Potter, and J.L. Kreider. 1981. A condition score relationship to body fat content of mares during gestation and lactation. In: Proc. 7th Equine Nutr. Physiol. Soc. Conf., Warrenton, Virginia p 105-110.

Henson, F.M., C. Davenport, L. Butler, I. Moran, W.D. Shingleton, L.B. Jeffcott, and P.N. Schofield. 1997. Effects of insulin and insulin-like growth factors I and II on the growth of equine fetal and neonatal chondrocytes. Equine Vet. J. 29(6):441-447.

Jeffcott, L.B., and F.M. Henson. 1998. Studies on growth cartilage in the horse and their application to aetiopathogenesis of dyschondroplasia (osteochondrosis) Vet. J. 156(3):177-92.

Jenkins, D.J., T.M. Wolever, R.H. Taylor, H. Barker, H. Fielden, J.M. Baldwin, A.C. Bowling, H.C. Newman, A.L. Jenkins, and D.V. Goff. 1981. Glycemic index of foods: A physiological basis for carbohydrate exchange. Amer. J. Clin. Nutr. 34:362-366.

NRC. 1989. Nutrient Requirements of Horses (5th Ed.). National Academy Press, Washington, DC.

Pagan, J.D., R.J. Geor, S.E. Caddel, P.B. Pryor, and K.E. Hoekstra. 2001. The relationship between glycemic response and the incidence of OCD in thoroughbred weanlings: A field study. In: Proc. 17th Amer. Assoc. Equine Pract. Conv.

Pagan, J.D., S.G. Jackson, and S. Caddel. 1996. A summary of growth rates of thoroughbreds in Kentucky. Pferdeheilkunde 12:285-289.

Pawlak, D.B., J.M. Bryson, G.S. Denyer, and J.C. Brand-Miller. 2001. High glycemic index starch promotes hypersecretion of insulin and higher body fat in rats without affecting insulin sensitivity. J. Nutr.131:99-104.

Ralston, S.L. 1995. Postprandial hyperglycemica/hyperinsulinemia in young horses with osteochondritis dissecans lesions. J. Anim. Sci. 73:184 (Abstr.).

Differential diagnosis and nutritional management of equine exertional rhabdomyolysis

Stephanie Valberg
Large Animal Medicine, Department of Veterinary Population Medicine,
University of Minnesota, 1365 Gortner Ave, St Paul MN, USA

Summary

Exertional rhabdomyolysis (ER) has been recognized in horses for more than 100 years as a syndrome of muscle pain and cramping associated with exercise. Recently it has been recognized that this syndrome has numerous possible causes. Sporadic forms of ER are due to over-training and muscle strain, dietary deficiencies of electrolytes, vitamin E and selenium or exercise in conjunction with herpes or influenza virus infections. Chronic forms are due to specific inherited abnormalities such as polysaccharide storage myopathy (PSSM) in Quarter Horses, Warmbloods and Draft breeds or recurrent exertional rhabdomyolysis (RER) in Thoroughbreds, Standardbreds and Arabians. PSSM, a glycogen storage disorder, can effectively be managed by providing regular daily exercise and a high fiber diet with minimal starch and sugar and provision of a fat supplement. RER appears to be a disorder of intracellular calcium regulation that is triggered by excitement. Changing management to provide horses with a calm environment and training schedule and substitution of fat for grains in high caloric rations are helpful means to manage this condition.

Introduction

Exertional rhabdomyolysis has been recognized in horses for more than 100 years as a syndrome of muscle pain and cramping associated with exercise. Exertional rhabdomyolysis continues to be a performance-limiting or career-ending disorder for many equine athletes. In the last 15 years, research advances have provided greater insight into this syndrome. Of greatest importance is the realization that exertional rhabdomyolysis comprises several myopathies that, despite similarities in clinical presentation, differ considerably in regards to pathogenesis (cellular events, reactions, and other pathologic mechanisms occurring in the development of disease) (Valberg *et al.*, 1999a). In addition, new knowledge regarding effective management of horses with exertional rhabdomyolysis, particularly with regard to diet, has significantly reduced the severity ER in many horses.

Clinical signs of Exertional Rhabdomyolysis

Clinical signs of exertional rhabdomyolysis usually occur shortly after the beginning of exercise. The most common sign is firm and painful muscles over the lumbar (loin) and sacral (croup) regions of the topline, including the large gluteal muscles (Firshman 2003). Excessive sweating, quick, shallow breathing, rapid heart rate, and muscle tremors are also noticed. In extreme cases, horses may be reluctant or refuse to move and may produce discolored urine due to the release of myoglobin from damaged muscle tissue. Episodes of ER vary from subclinical to severe in which massive muscle necrosis and renal failure from myoglobinuria occurs.

Diagnosis of Exertional Rhabdomyolysis

In order to confirm a diagnosis of ER blood samples should be obtained to determine that serum creatine kinase (CK) and aspartate transaminase (AST) activity are elevated. When muscle cells are damaged, CK and AST are released into the bloodstream within hours. AST activity may be heightened in asymptomatic horses with chronic exertional rhabdomyolysis.

Muscle biopsies are helpful in distinguishing various forms of chronic tying-up. Biopsies taken at our veterinary hospital are from the middle gluteal muscle using a 6 mm modified Bergstrom biopsy needle and frozen immediately. Biopsies shipped by referring veterinarians to our laboratory are of the semimembranosus/ semitendinosus muscles performed by an open surgical technique (see http://www.academic-server.cvm.umn.edu/neuromuscularlab/Home.htm for more information). Muscle biopsies are stained with a battery of histochemical and tinctorial stains and examined under the microscope to look for specific types of exertional rhabdomyolysis.

Classification

Exertional rhabdomyolysis can be subdivided into one of two distinct forms - sporadic and chronic. Horses that experience a single episode or infrequent episodes of muscle necrosis with exercise are categorized as having sporadic exertional rhabdomyolysis, whereas horses that have repeated episodes of exertional rhabdomyolysis accompanied by increased muscle enzyme activity, even with mild exertion, are classified as having chronic exertional rhabdomyolysis.

Sporadic exertional rhabdomyolysis

Sporadic exertional rhabdomyolysis occurs most commonly in horses that are exercised in excess of their level of conditioning. This happens frequently when a training program is accelerated too abruptly, particularly after an idle period of a few days, weeks, or months. Endurance competitions held on hot, humid days may elicit sporadic exertional rhabdomyolysis in susceptible horses because of high body temperatures, loss of fluid and electrolytes in sweat, and depletion of muscle energy stores. These metabolic imbalances can lead to muscle dysfunction and damage. In some instances, horses seem more prone to exertional rhabdomyolysis following respiratory infections. Therefore, horses should not be exercised if they have a fever, cough, nasal discharge, or other signs of respiratory compromise.

Nutritional management of sporadic exertional rhabdomyolysis

A well-designed exercise program and a nutritionally balanced diet with appropriate caloric intake and adequate vitamins and minerals are the core elements of treating exertional rhabdomyolysis. In some cases, deficiencies of vitamins, minerals or electrolytes may cause signs of muscle pain and stiffness in horses. Suggested deficiencies include:

Vitamin E and selenium

Adequate amounts of vitamin E and selenium prevent the detrimental interaction of peroxides with lipid membranes of the muscle cell. Most horses with chronic rhabdomyolysis have adequate or more than adequate concentrations of vitamin E and selenium, and further supplementation has not been found to have protective effects on muscle integrity in exercising horses (Roneus 1985). Many feeds, particularly those designed for horses with rhabdomyolysis, provide adequate selenium supplementation and caution should be taken not to provide excessive selenium in the diet. Likewise, sufficient vitamin E is provided in most diets by green grasses, well-cured hay, and rice bran. The new natural vitamin E products that consist of water-soluble particles appear to be better absorbed than synthetic vitamin E.

Electrolytes and minerals

Horses performing in hot weather often develop electrolyte imbalances, particularly if exercise continues for several hours. Free-choice access to loose salt or a salt block should be provided to these horses, or alternatively, one to four ounces of salt can be added to the feed daily. Extreme climatic conditions may necessitate the use of commercial electrolyte mixtures containing a 2:1:4 ratio of sodium:potassium:chloride. Fresh water should be available to horses at all times, especially if they are being supplemented with electrolytes.

Dietary imbalances of electrolytes, particularly deficiencies of sodium, potassium, and calcium, have been implicated in exertional rhabdomyolysis (Harris 1991). Correction of imbalances may be crucial in the management of some exertional rhabdomyolysis cases.

Chromium

Supplementation with oral chromium (5 mg/day) has been suggested to calm horses and improve their responses to exercise possibly by affecting glucose and glycogen metabolism, possibly by potentiating the action of insulin (Ott 1999). The purported calming effect of chromium may be beneficial in horses with recurrent exertional rhabdomyolysis because it appears that stress is a critical precipitator of this disorder. However, because PSSM horses display abnormal sensitivity to insulin, chromium supplementation may be counterproductive in these animals.

Chronic Exertional Rhabdomyolysis

Chronic exertional rhabdomyolysis arises frequently from heritable myopathies such as polysaccharide storage myopathy (PSSM) or recurrent exertional rhabdomyolysis (RER). Other causes of chronic exertional rhabdomyolysis are probable; however, their etiopathologies remain unknown.

Recurrent Exertional Rhabdomyolysis (RER)

Recurrent exertional rhabdomyolysis commonly afflicts Thoroughbreds and likely Standardbreds and Arabians (Beech *et al.*, 1993, 1994). During a racing season, 5-10 % of Thoroughbreds often exhibit signs of RER and of those 2 and 3 year-old horses with RER, up to 15% may not be able to train sufficiently to race at all that season (MacLeay *et al.*, 1999a). Interestingly, if horses that experience RER can race, there is no difference between their performances and those of matched control horses. In one investigation of heritability, a farm had 18 horses tie-up repeatedly over three years. Fourteen of the broodmares on this farm were bred to a particular stallion; all of the offspring experienced tying-up. When the same mares were bred to another stallion, only two of the offspring tied-up. On a different farm, one mare prone to tying-up produced six offspring with the disorder. A breeding trial conducted at the University of Minnesota as well as pedigree studies from a variety of farms now suggest that susceptibility to RER is inherited as an autosomal dominant trait (MacLeay *et al.*, 1999b). Studies in Standardbred horses also suggest that there is a heritable basis for this condition (Collinder *et al.*, 1997).

The most severely affected horses are nervous young (two-year-old) fillies in race training at tracks. The sex predilection for females, however, is not obvious in older horses with RER. Episodes of RER occur most often when horses are restrained during exercise, and incidences of RER may become more frequent as level of fitness increases. Clinical expression of RER is often stress-induced, and horses with RER are typically described as having nervous or very nervous temperaments. Older horses with RER may have muscle stiffness and soreness but only show overt evidence of tying-up after Steeplechase or cross-country phases of a 3 day event.

A specific cause for RER in Thoroughbreds has recently been identified (Lentz *et al.*, 1999, Lentz 2002). It appears that the mechanism by which muscle contraction is regulated can be disrupted by excitement and exercise in some susceptible horses. This discovery was based on the observation that intercostal muscle biopsies from RER horses readily develop contractures when exposed to agents (halothane and caffeine) that increase intramuscular calcium release. The threshold for developing a contracture is much lower for RER horses compared to normal horses similar to a muscle disease in people and swine called malignant hyperthermia. Every time a muscle contracts, calcium is released from muscle storage sites and then taken back up into storage sites for muscle relaxation. The altered contraction and relaxation of muscle suggests that abnormal intracellular calcium regulation is the cause of this form of RER. These intramuscular calcium concentrations are extremely small compared to the amount of calcium in the rest of the body and are completely independent of dietary calcium concentrations.

Diet manipulation is becoming the method of choice in controlling RER, particularly in equine athletes that are closely monitored for pharmacological substances. A well-designed exercise program and a nutritionally balanced diet with appropriate caloric intake and adequate vitamins and minerals are the core elements of treating RER.

Effect of modulation of dietary fat and starch

Increasing dietary fat supplementation and decreasing dietary starch have resulted in beneficial effects to horses with RER, however, the mechanism for this is not clearly understood (Valentine *et al.*, 1998, MacLeay *et al.*, 2000, McKenzie *et al.*, 2003a, 2003b). Fat supplementation is only beneficial to RER horses when total dietary caloric intake is high. The beneficial effects of fat supplementation in RER horses may be due to the exclusion of dietary starch rather than specific protective effects of high dietary fat. Given the close relationship between nervousness and tying-up in horses with RER, avoiding anxiety and excitability by reducing dietary starch and increasing dietary fat may decrease predisposition to RER by making these horses calmer prior to exercise.

Controlled and field studies have shown that feeding 2 to 5 pounds of rice bran or rice bran-based products (Re-Leve by Hallway Feeds, Lexington, KY) to both PSSM and RER horses has resulted in significant improvement in disease (McKenzie *et al.*, 2003b).

Recommended diets for horses with RER

As with any horse, feeding forage at a rate of 1.5-2% of body weight is a fundamental part of the diet. RER horses seem to benefit from fat supplementation only when they require high caloric intakes. Once caloric needs are assessed, a diet should be designed with an appropriate amount of fat and starch. Thoroughbred horses with frequent episodes of rhabdomyolysis are usually being fed 5-15 pounds of sweet feed per day. The incidence of subclinical rhabdomyolysis is low in Thoroughbreds being fed a moderate caloric intake whether it is in the form of sweet feed or rice bran. However, when calories are increased by the addition of more sweet feed, the incidence of subclinical and clinical rhabdomyolysis is much greater. One way to lower serum CK after exercise when a high caloric intake is required is to feed a low-starch, high-fat ration. For RER horses, the recommendation is to feed no greater than 20% of daily DE as nonstructural carbohydrate and to supply 20-25% of daily DE from fat. The diet should contain no more than five pounds of sweet feed, 600 ml of vegetable oil, and five pounds of rice bran per day. For horses undergoing intense exercise, the combination of sweet feed and oil or sweet feed and rice bran does not achieve an adequate DE without feeding amounts of cereal grains that have been shown to elicit rhabdomyolysis in susceptible horses.

A specialized diet, Re-Leve, (www.Re-Leve.com) has been designed for intensely exercised horses with chronic exertional rhabdomyolysis. Re-Leve contains 13% fat by weight or 20% DE as fat and only 9% DE as starch. In the USA, ReLeve is formulated to include rice bran, whereas in Europe, rice bran is not included in the formulation for ReLeve because rice bran is considered to be a performance enhancing substance in countries such as the UK. This type of high-energy diet for RER horses might be provided through a combination of other commercially available grains, several fat supplements, and highly fermentable fiber sources (soy hulls, beet pulp). Other commercially available concentrates contain moderate amounts of fat (6-10%) and have lower NSC values (17-30 % by weight). However, they cannot be fed in the quantities necessary to achieve the calories required to sustain intense exercise in RER horses without exceeding recommended NSC limits for these horses. They should therefore be combined with a fat supplement.

All supplemental feeds should be reduced in amount on days when energy requirements are not as high, particularly if the horse is at risk of weight gain. Other management strategies may help to decrease the intensity of the postprandial glycemic response, and include feeding small meals, providing at least 1.5-2.0% body weight per day in forage, and feeding a forage source either two hours before or concurrently with any grain. Avoiding high starch supplements such as molasses is also important.

Surprisingly, recent studies in RER horses show that significant reductions or normalization of post-exercise serum CK activity occurs within a week of commencing a diet providing 20% DE as fat and 9% DE as starch. This low serum CK activity compared to the high CK activity observed in the same horses on an isocaloric diet where 40% DE was starch was not the result of any measurable change in muscle glycogen or metabolism during exercise. Potentially, the rapid response to decreasing starch and increasing fat was a result of neurohormonal changes that resulted in a calmer demeanor, lower pre-exercise heart rates, and a decreased incidence of stress-induced rhabdomyolysis. Avoiding prolonged stall rest in fit Thoroughbreds with RER is also important since post-exercise CK activity is higher following two days of rest compared to values taken later in the week when performing consecutive days of the same amount of submaximal exercise. It is quite possible that exercise exerts beneficial effects on horses with chronic exertional rhabdomyolysis that are separate from the impact of reduction in dietary starch and/or fat supplementation. Failure to implement an appropriate exercise routine will likely lead to failure to control rhabdomyolysis.

Additional management strategies for chronic exertional rhabdomyolysis

RER horses are often very fit when they develop rhabdomyolysis and require only a few days off before commencing a reduced amount of training. Stall confinement should be kept to less than 24 hours if possible. Since RER appears to be a stress-related disorder, management strategies to reduce stress and excitability in these horses are important. These include turn-out, exercising or feeding these horses before other horses, providing compatible equine company, and the judicious use of low-dose tranquilizers during training. Anecdotal reports of increased nervousness have been received when selenium is supplemented at higher than the recommended levels. Feeds designed for RER should be evaluated for their selenium concentrations and should not be supplemented in addition if adequate levels are provided in the feed.

Dantrolene (4mg/kg PO) given 1 hour before exercise to horses that are not fed their morning feed is effective in preventing RER (McKenzie et al., 2004). However, little absorption of dantrolene occurs in horses that have been on full feed at the time of administration. Dantrolene is used to prevent malignant hyperthermia in humans and swine by decreasing the release of calcium from the calcium release channel. Phenytoin (1.4-2.7 mg/kg PO BID), has also been advocated as a treatment for horses with RER (Beech 1988). Therapeutic levels vary, so oral doses are adjusted by monitoring serum levels to achieve 8 ug/ml and not exceed 12 ug/ml. Phenytoin acts on a number of ion channels within muscle and nerves including sodium and calcium channels. Unfortunately long-term treatment with dantrolene or phenytoin is expensive.

Polysaccharide Storage Myopathy (PSSM)

Polysaccharide storage myopathy affects primarily Quarter Horses and horses with Quarter Horse bloodlines such as Paints and Appaloosa (Valberg et al., 1992, 1997). In addition, Drafts, Warmbloods as well as Morgans have been diagnosed with this disorder. Horses with PSSM typically have calm dispositions and are in good body condition (Firshman et al., 2003). A change in exercise routine often triggers an episode of rhabdomyolysis. This change need not be profound; something as subtle and seemingly harmless as unaccustomed stall confinement may provoke an episode. Signs of PSSM include sweating, stretching out as if posturing to urinate, muscle fasciculations, and rolling or pawing following exercise. Severe cases may display stiffness and hesitance to move within minutes of starting exercise, and extreme cases may result in the horse being unable to stand and in discomfort even when lying down. Serum creatine kinase (CK) activity may be persistently elevated despite an extended period of rest.

Table 1. Feeding recommendations for an average-sized horse (500 kg) with Recurrent Exertional Rhabdomyolysis at varying levels of exertion.

	Maintenance	Light exercise	Moderate exercise	Intense exercise
Digestible Energy (Mcal/day)	16.4	20.5	24.6	32.8
% DE as NSC	<20%	<20%	<20%	<20%
% DE as fat	15%	15%	15%-20%	20-25%
Forage % bwt	1.5- 2.0 %	1.5- 2.0 %	1.5- 2.0 %	1.5- 2.0 %
Protein (grams/day)	697	767	836	906
Calcium (g)	30	33	36	39
Phosphorus (g)	20	22	24	26
Sodium (g)	22.5	33.5	33.8	41.3
Chloride (g)	33.8	50.3	50.6	62
Potassium (g)	52.5	78.3	78.8	96.4
Selenium (mg)	1.88	2.2	2.81	3.13
Vitamin E (IU)	375	700	900	1000

Daily requirements derived from multiple research studies (% NSC and % fat) and Kentucky Equine Research recommendations. NSC = Non Structural Carbohydrates
From: From: McKenzie et al., 2003a.

The muscle biopsy is very useful for identifying PSSM. PSSM is a glycogen storage disorder characterized by the accumulation of glycogen and abnormal polysaccharide complexes in 1-40% of skeletal muscle fibers (Valberg et al., 1992, Annandale et al., 2004). Muscle glycogen concentrations in affected horses are 1.5 to 4 times greater than in normal horses. In humans, glycogen storage diseases commonly result from impaired utilization and breakdown of glycogen by tissues. No limitations in the ability of skeletal muscle to metabolize glycogen have been identified in PSSM horses and in fact, PSSM horses have higher glycogen utilization rates than healthy horses during anaerobic exercise (Valberg et al., 1999). As such the metabolic defect responsible for marked glycogen accumulation appears to involve abnormal regulation of glycogen synthesis rather than a defect in utilization. We have found that horses with PSSM clear glucose from the bloodstream after an IV bolus, or oral meal much faster than normal horses (DeLaCorte et al., 1999a). It appears they do this because of increased

Table 2. *Potential rations for a 500-kg horse with Exertional Rhabdomyolysis.*

	Light exercise	Moderate exercise	Intense exercise
Forage Plus:	7-9 kg quality grass hay or pasture	7-9 kg quality grass hay or pasture	7-9 kg quality grass hay or 20:80 mix alfalfa/grass
Diet 1:*	1 kg sweet feed + 1 kg rice bran	2 kg sweet feed + 1 kg of rice bran	2.1 kg sweet feed + 1.4 kg of rice bran + 1.4 kg beet pulp**
or: Diet 2:	1.5 kg of Re-Leve	3 kg of Re-Leve	5 kg of Re-Leve
or: Diet 3:*	1 kg of sweet feed + 200 ml oil	2 kg of sweet feed + 500 ml oil	Combination cannot achieve required DE intake

*Vitamin and mineral supplement required for nonfortified feeds. The mineral recommended for the specific rice bran product should be provided (not necessary for Re-Leve).
**Soak beet pulp before feeding.
Addition of 50-100 g of salt per day to all rations is recommended based on level of exertion.
From: McKenzie *et al.*, 2003a.

insulin sensitivity. When insulin is given to PSSM horses it causes a profound drop in blood sugar, which lasts for twice as long relative to normal horses. Thus it appears that one of the abnormalities in PSSM is that when fed a starch meal, these horses, store a higher proportion of the absorbed glucose in their muscle compared to normal horses. The mechanism of glucose transport into muscles of PSSM does not appear to be regulated in the same fashion as healthy horses (Annandale *et al.*, 2004). Why this in itself causes muscle cells to become damaged with exercise is not clear at this time. Recent studies of single muscle fibers from PSSM horses obtained after light exercise show a much higher accumulation of IMP than in healthy horses. IMP normally only accumulates in muscle after strenuous exercise and is an indicator that there is a disruption in normal energy flux in PSSM muscle (Annandale 2005). Although the specific cause of PSSM in horses remains unknown, it can naively be seen as the opposite of type 2 Diabetes.

PSSM appears to be an inherited disorder, with recent evidence supporting a dominant rather than a recessive mode of inheritance (Valberg *et al.*, 1996,unpublished data). The development of rhabdomyolysis can occur in young foals and may precede the accumulation of abnormal polysaccharide in skeletal muscle (DeLaCorte *et al.*, 2002). Breeding of a horse with PSSM may well result in 50% of the offspring being affected regardless of the sire or dam chosen as a breeding partner. Expression of the disease may be impacted by the amount of exercise and dietary starch fed to young growing horses.

A glycogen storage disorder with similar histological characteristics occurs in draft breeds. Belgian and Percheron horses appear to have about a 35% prevalence of EPSM in the population (Valentine *et al.*, 2001, Firshman 2005). This syndrome is referred to as equine polysaccharide storage myopathy (EPSM). While similarities exist between PSSM and EPSM, draft horses with EPSM often exhibit signs not indicative of PSSM, including normal serum creatine kinase, difficulty backing and holding up limbs, a shivers-like gait, and loss of muscle mass. Some drafts afflicted with EPSM also show recumbency and weakness with only slight increases in serum CK and AST, and this combination of signs is not seen in Quarter horses with PSSM.

Prevention of Rhabdomyolysis with PSSM

Training: Horses with PSSM will **not** improve if the only change made is the addition of dietary fat (Valberg *et al.*, 1997, De La Corte *et al.*, 1999b). Prevention of further episodes of rhabdomyolysis requires a very gradual increase in the amount of daily exercise horses experience. Minimizing stress, providing regular routines and daily exercise are highly beneficial. Turn-out each day with other horses in as large an area as possible will keep the horse active and is in my experience the single most important thing that can benefit these horses. If there has been a recent severe episode of tying-up I recommend turning the horse out for 2 weeks on the diet recommended below. After switching your horse's diet for 2 weeks, horses can begin longing once a day for 5 minutes at a walk and trot. Gradually increase the time by 2 minutes a day. If the horse seems stiff, stand the horse still for 1 minute and see if the stiffness persists when walking. If stiffness is present, stop there, if not continue after a 2 minutes walk. When the horse can do 15 minutes provide a 5 minute break at a walk and gradually increase walking and trotting after this. Once the horse has reached 30 minutes of trotting on a lunge-line (with a break at 15 min) then I would begin to ride for 20 to 30 minutes and gradually increase the length and intensity of exercise. It should take at least 3 weeks before the horse is ridden. Keeping horses with PSSM fit increases oxidative metabolism, increases glycogen utilization and this seems the best prevention against further episodes of tying-up (Ribeiro 2004).

Dietary management of PSSM

As with any horse, feeding forage at a rate of 1.5-2% of body weight is a fundamental part of the diet. Once caloric needs are assessed, a diet should be designed with an appropriate amount of fat and starch. The amount of fat supplied to horses with PSSM is controversial. If PSSM horses are exercised regularly, many respond to low-calorie, low-starch diets that are only lightly supplemented with fat (Ribeiro 2004). Although recommended in the lay-press, most horses with exertional rhabdomyolysis do not require diets in which 25% of daily caloric intake is supplied by fat. In fact, such a diet is not always appropriate, is difficult to achieve in the face of high-calorie requirements, and may result in problems with weight gain and unpalatable diets.

Fat sources

Animal- and vegetable-based fats are the major sources of fat available for equine consumption. Examples of vegetable oils used for supplementation include corn, soy, peanut, coconut, safflower, linseed, flaxseed, and canola. Corn and soy oils are the most palatable. Vegetable oils are highly digestible (90-100%) and energy dense. While it can be messy to dole out, unpalatable to some horses, prone to rancidity in warm weather, and difficult to feed in large amounts, oil is an effective way to boost daily energy intake and may be the most economical way of providing fat to horses that do not require large amounts of supplementation. Horses receiving large amounts of oil may need vitamin E supplementation. Animal fat varies in digestibility (75-90%). Because animal fat is more saturated, it tends to be solid at room temperature and would need to be melted before being top-dressed on feed. Most horses find animal-based fats less palatable than vegetable-based fats. Rice bran contains about 20% fat as well as a considerable amount of vitamin E. Products containing rice bran are readily accepted by most horses. Commercial rice bran products are usually in powder or pellet form and are considerably more stable than animal fat and vegetable oils. Many rice bran-based products are balanced for calcium and phosphorus or are concurrently fed with a mineral supplement to offset the naturally high phosphorus content. Recently commercial diets have been developed for horses with exertional rhabdomyolysis. To be effective these diets need to be low in starch as well as high in fat.

Recommended diets for PSSM horses

In Quarter Horse-related breeds, PSSM can usually be managed with grass hay or mixed hay and a fat supplement that is balanced for vitamins and minerals. Starch should be decreased to less than 10% of daily digestible energy (DE) intake by eliminating grain and molasses. Rice bran can be gradually introduced into the diet as powder or as a pelleted feed. Some horses that will not eat powder will consume pelleted forms of rice bran. It is important for owners to understand that if horses eat the rice bran at a slower rate than sweet feed this can be beneficial as it reduces rapid absorption of starch. Depending on the caloric requirements of the horse, 1-5 pounds of rice bran can be fed but must be combined with a reduction in dietary starch to less than 10% of DE. Interestingly, rice bran oil is now being used as a means to manage human beings with type I and type II diabetes as it significantly lowers daily blood glucose concentrations (measured as glycosylated hemoglobin). Horses with severe forms of PSSM respond with lower serum CK activity when fed ReLeve compared to other rice bran products, likely due to the lower starch content of ReLeve compared to rice bran (Ribeiro *et al.*, 2004). In the USA, ReLeve is formulated to include rice bran, whereas in Europe, rice bran is not included in the formulation for ReLeve because rice bran is considered to be a performance enhancing substance in countries such as the UK. There are several palatable feeds available for horses that are high in fat. It is important to determine from the manufacturer which of the feeds also has less than 20% or ideally 10% NSC to be suitable for PSSM horses.

An alternative source of fat is corn oil added to alfalfa pellets. An upper limit of 600 ml of oil per day is recommended, and additional vitamin E should be added to the diet. It is not possible to achieve the high caloric requirements for intense exercise using oil supplementation of alfalfa pellets, sweet feed, or rice bran without exceeding recommended maximum amounts of these products. To achieve the appropriate caloric intake for PSSM horses performing intense exercise, high-fat, low-starch pelleted feeds designed for PSSM horses in intense exercise are recommended. Supplying fat at 6-10% by weight (or 15-20% of DE) of the entire ration to PSSM Quarter Horses (unless a higher energy intake is required for exercise) is likely quite sufficient for managing PSSM and further benefit from more fat has not been demonstrated in controlled trials. Note, however, that none of these diets will result in clinical improvement of muscle stiffness and exercise tolerance without gradually increasing the amount of daily exercise and maximizing access to turn-out.

Expectations of fat supplementation

The time required for improvement in signs of exertional rhabdomyolysis is controversial. It has been suggested that a minimum of four months of supplementation is required and that relapses are associated primarily with disruption of supplementation (Valentine

Table 3. feeding recommendations for an average-sized horse (500 kg) with PSSM at varying levels of exertion.

	Maintenance	Light exercise	Moderate exercise	Intense exercise
Digestible energy (Mcal/day)	16.4	20.5	24.6	32.8
% DE as NSC	<10%	<10%	<10%	<10%
% DE as fat	20%	20%	15%-20%	15%-20%
Forage % bwt	1.5- 2.0 %	1.5- 2.0 %	1.5- 2.0 %	1.5- 2.0 %
Protein (grams/day)	697	767	836	906
Calcium (g)	30	33	36	39
Phosphorus (g)	20	22	24	26
Sodium (g)	22.5	33.5	33.8	41.3
Chloride (g)	33.8	50.3	50.6	62
Potassium (g)	52.5	78.3	78.8	96.4
Selenium (mg)	1.88	2.2	2.81	3.13
Vitamin E (IU)	375	700	900	1000

Daily requirements derived from multiple research studies (% NSC and % fat) and Kentucky Equine Research recommendations. From: McKenzie et al., 2003a.

2001). However, in the author's experience clinical improvement with PSSM is more dependent on the amount of daily exercise and turn-out than on the length or amount of dietary fat supplementation. For example, when serum CK was monitored daily post-exercise, levels were almost within the normal range after four weeks of daily exercise, without fat supplementation (Valberg 1997). In addition, when PSSM horses were turned out 24 hours a day on grass, post-exercise serum CK was normal compared to high activities during the same exercise test with stall-kept horses on a hay diet. Thus, it seems that consistent fat supplementation without implementing a structured daily exercise regime in PSSM horses is highly likely to result in failure and confinement, while consuming high levels of fat is likely to lead to obesity.

Table 4. Potential rations for a 500-kg horse with Polysaccharide Storage Myopathy.

	Light exercise	Moderate exercise	Intense exercise
FORAGE PLUS:	7-9 kg quality grass hay or pasture	7-9 kg quality grass hay or pasture	7-9 kg quality grass hay or 20:80 mix alfalfa/grass
DIET 1*	1.5 kg rice bran	2.25 kg rice bran	Cannot achieve required DE intake with rice bran alone
DIET 2	1.5 kg Re-Leve	2.5 kg Re-Leve	5 kg of Re-Leve
DIET 3*	1.8 kg alfalfa pellets + 475 ml oil	Combination cannot achieve required DE intake	Combination cannot achieve required DE intake

*Vitamin and mineral supplement required for nonfortified feeds. The mineral recommended for the specific rice bran product should be provided (not necessary for Re-Leve).
Addition of 50-100 g of salt per day to all rations is recommended based on level of exertion.
From: McKenzie et al., 2003a.

References

Annandale, E.J., S.J. Valberg J.R. Mickelson and E.R. Seaquist. 2004. Insulin sensitivity and skeletal muscle glucose transport in Equine Polysaccharide Storage Myopathy. Neuromusc. Disorders 14:666-674.

Annandale EJ, Valberg SJ, Essen Gustavsson B The effect of submaximal exercise on adenine nucleotide concentrations in skeletal muscle fibers of horses with polysaccharide storage Myopathy Am J Vet Res 2005;66:839-845

Beech, J. 1994. Treating and preventing chronic intermittent rhabdomyolysis. Vet. Med. 458-461.

Beech, J., J.E. Fletcher, F. Lizzo, J. Johnston. 1988. Effect of phenytoin on the clinical signs and in vitro muscle twitch characteristics in horses with chronic intermittent rhabdomyolysis and myotonia, Am. J. Vet. Res. 49:2130-2133,

Beech, J., S. Lindborg, J.E. Fletcher, F. Lizzo, L.Tripolitis and K. Braund. 1993. Caffeine contractures, twitch characteristics and the threshold for Ca^{2+}-induced Ca^{2+} release in skeletal muscle from horses with chronic intermittent rhabdomyolysis. Res. Vet. Sci. 54:110.

Collinder, E., A. Lindholm and M. Rasmuson. 1997. Genetic markers in standardbred trotters susceptible to the rhabdomyolysis syndrome. Equine Vet J. 29:117-120.

De La Corte, F.D., S.J. Valberg, S. Williamson, J.M. MacLeay and J.R. Mickelson. 1999a. Enhanced glucose uptake in horses with polysaccharide storage myopathy (PSSM). Am. J. Vet. Res. 60:458-462.

De La Corte, F.D., S.J. Valberg, S. Williamson, J.M. MacLeay and J.R. Mickelson. 1999b. The effect of feeding a fat supplement to horses with polysaccharide storage myopathy. World Equine Veterinary Review Vol. 4.No.2:12-19.

DeLaCorte, F.D., S.J. Valberg, J.M. MacLeay and J.R. Mickelson. 2002. Developmental onset of polysaccharide storage myopathy in 4 Quarter Horse foals. J. Vet. Int. Med. 16:581-587.

Firshman, A.M., S.J. Valberg, J. Bender and C. Finno. 2003. Epidemiologic characteristics and management of polysaccharide storage myopathy in Quarter Horses. Am. J. Vet. Res. 64:1319-1327.

Firshman AM, Valberg SJ, Karges TL, Benedict LE, Annandale EJ, Seaquist ER. Serum Creatine Kinase Response to Exercise During Dexamethasone-induced Insulin Resistance in Four Quarter Horses with Polysaccharide Storage Myopathy. Am J Vet Res (in press)

Firshman AM, Baird JD and Valberg SJ. A Prospective Study .of Polysaccharide Storage Myopathy and Shivers in Belgian Draft Horses J Vet Med Assoc (in press).

Harris PA and Snow DH. Role of electrolyte imbalances in the pathophysiology of the equine rhabdomyolysis syndrome. 1991 In: *Equine Exercise Physiology* 3 ed. SGB Persson, A Lindholm and LB Jeffcott. ICEEP Publications, Davis CA, pp 435.

Lentz, L.R., S.J. Valberg, E. Balog, J.R. Mickelson and E.M. Gallant. 1999. Abnormal regulation of contraction in equine recurrent exertional rhabdomyolysis. Am. J. Vet. Res. 60:992-999.

Lentz LR, Valberg SJ, Herold L, Onan GW, Mickelson JR and Gallant EM. 2002. Myoplasmic calcium regulation in myotubes from horses with recurrent exertional rhabdomyolysis Am J Vet Res;63:1724-1731.

MacLeay, J.M., S.J. Valberg, C.J. Geyer., S.A. Sorum and M.D. Sorum. 1999a Epidemiological factors influencing exertional rhabdomyolysis in Thoroughbred racehorses. Am. J. Vet. Res. 60:1562-1566.

MacLeay, J.M., S.J. Valberg, C.J. Geyer., S.A. Sorum and M.D. Sorum. 1999b. Heritable basis for recurrent exertional rhabdomyolysis in thoroughbred racehorses. Am. J. Vet. Res. 60:250-256.

MacLeay, J.M., S.J. Valberg, J. Pagan, J.A. Billstrom and J Roberts. 2000. Effect of diet and exercise intensity on serum CK activity in Thoroughbreds with recurrent exertional rhabdomyolysis. Am. J. Vet. Res. 61:1390-1395.

McKenzie, E.M., S.J. and Valberg J. Pagan. 2003a. Nutritional management of exertional rhabdomyolysis. Pages 727-734. In: Current Therapy in Equine Veterinary Medicine 5. Robinson, N.E. (ed.). Saunders, St Louis, MO.

McKenzie, E.C., S.J. Valberg, S. Godden, J.D. Pagan, J.M. MacLeay, R.J. Geor and G.P. Carlson. 2003b. Effect of dietary starch, fat and bicarbonate content on exercise responses and serum creatine kinase activity in equine recurrent exertional rhabdomyolysis. J. Vet. Int. Med. 17:693-701.

McKenzie, E.C., S.J. Valberg, S.M. Godden and C.J. Finno. 2004. The effect of oral dantrolene sodium on post-exercise serum creatine kinase activity in thoroughbred horses with recurrent exertional rhabdomyolysis. Am. J. Vet. Res. 65:74-79.

Ott EA, Kivipelto J. 1999. Influence of chromium tripicolinate on growth and glucose metabolism in yearling horses. J Anim Sci.;77(11):3022-30.

Ribeiro, W., S.J. Valberg, J.D. Pagan and E. B. Gustavsson. 2004. The effect of varying dietary starch and fat content on creatine kinase activity and substrate availability in equine polysaccharide storage myopathy. J. Vet. Int.Med.18:887-894.

Roneus B and Hakkarainen J. 1985. Vitamin E in skeletal muscle tissue and blood glutathione peroxidase activity from horses with azoturia-tying-up syndrome. *Acta Vet Scand*;26:425-428.

Valberg, S., G.H. Cardinet III, G.P. Carlson and S. DiMauro. 1992. Polysaccharide storage myopathy associated with exertional rhabdomyolysis in the horse. Neuromusc. Disorders 2:351-359.

Valberg, S.J., C. Geyer, S.A. Sorum and G.H. Cardinet III. 1996. Familial basis for exertional rhabdomyolysis in Quarter Horse-related breeds. Amer. J. Vet. Res. 57:286-290.

Valberg, S.J., J.M. MacLeay and J.R. Mickelson. 1997. Polysaccharide storage myopathy associated with exertional rhabdomyolysis in horses. Comp. Cont. Educ. 19(9):1077-1086.

Valberg, S.J., J.M. MacLeay, J.A. Billstrom, M.A. Hower-Moritz and J.R. Mickelson. 1999. Skeletal muscle metabolic response to exercise in horses with polysaccharide storage myopathy. Equine Vet. J. 31:43-47.

Valberg, S.J., J.R. Mickelson, E.M. Gallant, J.M. MacLeay, L. Lentz and F.D. De La Corte. 1999. Exertional rhabdomyolysis in Quarter Horses and Thoroughbreds; one syndrome, multiple etiologies. International Conference on Equine Exercise Physiology. Equine Vet. J. Suppl. 30:533-538.

Valentine, B.A., H.F. Hintz, K.M. Freels, A.J. Reynolds and K.N. Thompson. 1998. Dietary control of exertional rhabdomyolysis in horses. J. Am. Vet. Med. Assoc. 212:1588-1593.

Valentine, B.A., R.J. Van Saun, K.N. Thompson and H.F. Hintz. 2001. Role of dietary carbohydrate and fat in horses with equine polysaccharide storage myopathy. J. Am. Vet. Med. Assn. 219:1537-1544.

Impact of diseases on the gastrointestinal microflora, nutritional prevention of these diseases and nutritional management after occurrence

Scott J. Weese
Dept of Clinical Studies, Ontario Veterinary College, University of Guelph,
Guelph, Ontario, Canada

Introduction

The equine intestinal tract contains a vast, complex and dynamic population of microorganisms that are necessary for health, and indeed, survival of the horse. At most times, the intestinal microflora is assumed to be a relatively stable population with endogenous controls ensuring a beneficial balance of organisms. However, changes in this microbial population can occur, both as a cause and result of disease. An understanding of the response of the gastrointestinal microflora to disease states would be useful to help prevent, lessen or correct adverse effects. Unfortunately, at this point, we have a very superficial understanding of the gastrointestinal microflora as a whole, with little specific information regarding the effects of different stressors and diseases. Bacterial culture is typically used to evaluate the intestinal microflora, however culture has serious limitations based on the complexity of the microflora; varying nutritional and environmental requirements of different bacteria (many of which are unknown); effects of sampling, handling and storage on bacterial recovery; the inability to culture many organisms, and the inability to identify a significant percentage of intestinal organisms. In humans, a recent study reported that the majority of bacterial sequences identified from the intestinal tract of healthy people were novel bacteria, demonstrating our poor overall knowledge of the normal human intestinal microflora (Eckburg et al., 2005). Further, based on information from other species it is highly likely that the intestinal microflora varies significantly between healthy horses, limiting our assessment of changes in the microflora. That being said, by evaluating information that is available regarding horses and extrapolating from information known about other species, some general assumptions and hypotheses can be made, and can potentially help with the management and prevention of intestinal microflora disruption while the equine microflora is being studied further.

Impact of disease on the gastrointestinal microflora

It is likely that diseases of virtually any body system can have effects on the gastrointestinal microflora. A few different mechanisms of disease-associated intestinal microflora disruption should be considered: changes from the specific disease process, changes occurring as a result of treatment, changes that develop from altered intestinal motility, changes that result from management changes associated with disease (withholding feed, diet changes, changes in exercise...) and exposure to different enteropathogens as a result of change in location (especially hospitalization). In many (or most) cases, these changes are probably mild and result in no recognizable adverse effects. However, clinical disease can occur, and in some cases can be severe or even fatal.

Disease specific changes

It is often difficult, if not impossible, to differentiate specific disease effects from those caused by intervention such as treatment and management changes. For some diseases, adverse effects on the intestinal microflora have been clearly demonstrated. Perhaps the most obvious (and most dramatic clinically) is colitis (severe diarrhea). Colitis is a serious problem in horses that typically results from overgrowth of one or more pathogenic bacteria in the intestinal tract. This can be from overgrowth of bacteria previously present in low levels in the intestinal tract, or from ingestion of new organisms. The overgrowth of pathogenic bacteria, with resulting changes in the intestinal environment, can produce dramatic changes in the intestinal microflora.

Similarly, grain overload involves a dramatic change in the intestinal microflora from over-ingestion of carbohydrates. Most types of colic are probably associated with microflora changes because of a combination of primary disease effects (ie altered intestinal motility) and changes associated with treatment (ie feed withdrawal). Any disease that affects appetite can be presumed to have some impact on the intestinal flora, with more severe changes probably occurring with longer duration of disease and when little or no food is ingested.

Effects of treatment

In some situations, it is human intervention, not the primary disease process, which causes an effect on the intestinal microflora. While many treatments or management changes that affect the microflora are unavoidable, it is important to understand the potential adverse effects so that they can be minimized.

One of the most recognized treatment factors affecting the intestinal microflora is administration of antimicrobials. Administration of any antimicrobial can be expected to have some impact on the intestinal microflora. The antimicrobial spectrum, drug level achieved in the intestinal tract, and the presence or absence of local antimicrobial inhibitors are all likely important in determining the risk of individual drugs. Horse-specific factors are probably equally important. These include the presence of potential pathogens (ie *Clostridium difficile, Salmonella*) at low levels in the intestinal tract and the composition of the remainder of the protective microflora. Variability of the microflora between horses could have an impact on the likelihood of disease. Additionally, exposure to enteropathogens from the environment, feed or other horses may play a role in the likelihood of disease. There may also be a role of geography, as it appears that the risk of development of antimicrobial-associated diarrhea from different drugs varies between regions. In particular, fatal *Clostridium difficile* colitis is a significant concern in mares whose foals are treated with erythromycin because of the potential for low dose erythromycin exposure (Baverud *et al.*, 1998). However, the same problems are uncommonly reported in other areas.

There have only been a few studies regarding effects of antimicrobials on the intestinal microflora. One study reported a 10-fold decrease in coliform counts following trimethoprim-sulfa treatment, but no other significant changes and the authors felt that overall no major changes had occurred (Gustafsson *et al.*, 1999). Another study reported large increases in coliforms, *Bacteroides* spp and streptococci, disappearance of *Veillonella* spp and appearance of *Clostridium perfringens* following oral administration of oxytetracycline, but not trimethoprim-sulfa (White and Prior, 1982).

While there is a common perception that oral administration of antimicrobials is at higher risk of causing microflora disruption, this is not necessarily true is all situations. After administration via any route, there will be varying degree of exposure of the intestinal microflora to the drug. Drugs such as tetracyclines that are excreted in bile may reach particularly high levels in the intestinal tract. It is clear that oral administration of many drugs is a high-risk situation in terms of the potential for development of colitis. However, there is no evidence that oral administration of antimicrobials *that are commonly used in horses* is more likely to cause colitis or other manifestations of microflora disruption than parenteral use. One study reported no difference in intestinal microflora changes between oral and intravenous administration of trimethoprim-sulfa in healthy horses.[3] Another study reported that oral administration of trimethoprim-sulfa did not predispose horses to development of diarrhea compared with other antimicrobials (Wilson *et al.*, 1996).

Another potential treatment associated impact on the intestinal microflora is the use of gastric ulcer treatment or prophylaxis. Drugs that affect gastric acidity, particularly proton pump inhibitors (ie omeprazole), might have an effect on the microflora. This is of particular concern in horses with other risk factors. The acidic environment of the stomach is an important barrier that helps kill ingested bacteria. In people, the use of proton pump inhibitors is highly associated with nosocomial (hospital-origin) *Clostridium difficile* diarrhea (Dial *et al.*, 2004), leading to calls to restrict the use of these drugs in hospitalized patients. While not specifically evaluated in horses, it is possible that anti-ulcer therapy could facilitate survival of ingested pathogens and increase the risk of flora disruption and disease.

Changes from altered intestinal motility

Changes in intestinal motility, either increased or decreased transit time, can potentially affect the microflora. The primary disease, withholding of feed, general anesthesia, certain drugs and pain, can all potentially affect motility. In one study, horses undergoing orthopedic surgery that did not receive phenylbutazone post-operatively were at risk for developing reduced fecal output (Little, Redding and Blikslager, 2001). It is possible that any type of pain, particularly severe and chronic pain such as is associated with certain orthopedic disorders, could negatively impact intestinal motility and thereby have adverse consequences on the intestinal microflora.

Pathogen exposure

Horses are continually exposed to a variety of pathogens in the environment, from contact with other horses and in feedstuffs. In most situations, pathogens are not present in sufficient numbers to cause disease. Environmental or feed-associated exposure to pathogens can become clinically relevant when high doses of pathogens are ingested and/or when concurrent risk factors such as are described above are present. Hospitalized horses must be considered at particular risk because of the potential for encountering infectious agents during hospitalization, the primary disease that necessitated hospitalization, and effects of treatments that may be present. The most commonly reported nosocomial intestinal pathogen in equine hospitals is *Salmonella*, and outbreaks of salmonellosis have been widely reported (Schott *et al.*, 2001; Van Duijkeren *et al.*, 1994).

Prevention of intestinal microflora disruption

Prevention of intestinal microflora disruption is impossible. Horses with no signs of any disease, on a constant diet, with no management changes or any other risk factor can still develop disease from intestinal microflora disruption. Our limited knowledge of the normal state and the dynamics involved in development of microflora disruption limits our ability to completely prevent disease. Indeed, it is possible that some degree of disruption occurs regularly from a variety of factors, but overt disease does not develop and the incident goes unrecognized. The main focus is *reducing* (not eliminating) the likelihood and incidence of clinically significant flora disruption.

Any horse with any illness should be considered at increased risk of disease arising from intestinal microflora disruption. Accordingly, steps should be taken to try to decrease exposure to potential pathogens and to limit the impact of any other associated risk factors. Antimicrobial therapy should only be used when absolutely required, and for the shortest duration possible. Only drugs that are known to be relatively safe in horses should be used. Newer antimicrobials, particularly oral drugs, should not be used until safety and efficacy have been assessed experimentally. Feed withholding and feed changes should be limited as much as possible. Any diet changes should be made gradually. Management changes should be kept to a minimum and unnecessary transportation should be avoided. Horses with potentially infectious gastrointestinal tract disease should be isolated and handled using standard barrier protocols, to prevent dissemination of pathogens on the farm or in the hospital. Cleaning, disinfection and other infection control measures should be reviewed to ensure that relevant pathogens are being adequately addressed (Dwyer, 2004).

Nutritional management after intestinal microflora disruption

There is essentially no objective information regarding specific management of animals with disruptions of the intestinal microflora, nor is there any easy way to identify such cases in the absence of overt signs such as diarrhea or colic.

Without objective evidence, recommendations can only be made based on our current (limited) understanding of the intestinal microflora and with extrapolation from other species. Care must be taken, however, when trying to directly apply information from most other species because of the unique nature of the intestinal tract in the horse. It is critical to remember that every horse may have somewhat different nutritional requirements and sensitivities. There is no such thing as a 'standard' feeding regimen that will work for all horses. Nutritional guidelines are only that; guidelines. They must be adapted to suit the specific horse.

The standard statement of "above all do not harm" should be considered when considering any potential measures to affect the intestinal microflora. Minor transient changes in the intestinal microflora are likely inconsequential and require no intervention. Intervention could be beneficial in cases with more serious changes that are associated with disease or a higher likelihood of development of disease. Ideally, these cases would be identified before serious disease developed, something that we are currently unable to do with any degree of confidence.

Likely the most important general nutritional approach to restoring the balanced microbial population in many cases is provision of a diet similar to that which would be encountered in the wild, or in other terms, a diet similar to that with which the intestinal tract evolved. The essence of this type of management is provision of good quality hay in reasonable levels, with an appropriate introduction period, and to permit the horse to eat during much of the day. Controlled pasture grazing could also be beneficial in horses that have been acclimated to grazing and where grazing is not contraindicated for other reasons (ie recurrent pasture-associated laminitis). Sudden access to pasture by a horse not accustomed to easy fresh grass should be avoided. While provision of a good quality roughage-based diet may be adequate in some situations, different or additional measures may be required at times. Also, specific diseases may necessitate different nutritional management. It is important to consider feeding in the broadest sense, trying to balance the pros and cons of different types of feeding to achieve the best overall feeding program.

Increased energy requirements may be present in some circumstances, particularly in horses with ongoing disease or those that have lost considerable weight because of the primary disease (ie colitis). However, care must be taken not to attempt to correct the situation too quickly or too early. Overly aggressive re-introduction of feeding, particularly concentrates, can have negative consequences. It is important to remember that a gradual return to normal body condition is ideal and that aggressive feeding of a convalescing horse may increase the likelihood of further problems developing. In some situations, the optimal diet may need to be sacrificed in order to ensure that the horse eats. In general, it is preferable for a horse to eat a suboptimal diet in the convalescent period versus no food. Therefore, if an ill or high-risk horse refuses the optimal diet, other reasonable but perhaps suboptimal diets should be offered.

Numerous nutritional supplements are available for use in horses, and many are marketed for prevention or treatment of intestinal microflora disruption. Predominant among these products are prebiotics, probiotics and synbiotics. Prebiotics are non-digestible food ingredients that beneficially affect the animal by stimulating growth and/or activity of certain intestinal bacteria. Typically, they are targeted at increasing the numbers of lactic acid bacteria, particularly *Lactobacillus* and *Bifidobacterium*. Prebiotics consist mainly of non-digestible fructooligosaccharides and soybean oligosaccharides. Not all potentially beneficial organisms can utilize all prebiotics and if an increase in a specific component in the intestinal microflora is desired, then testing is required to ensure that the target bacteria can actually utilize the selected prebiotic. Prebiotics that have been used in other species must be specifically tested in horses to determine whether the same beneficial effects occurs, and to ensure that growth of potentially pathogenic organisms does not occur. At this point, no prebiotics have been proven to be effective for treatment or prevention of disease in horses.

Probiotics are living microorganisms that, when ingested in certain numbers exert a beneficial effect beyond that of their nutritional value (Guarner and Schaafsma, 1998). Initial theories revolved around 'competitive exclusion' where 'good' bacteria eliminated or suppressed 'bad' bacteria. While competitive exclusion may play a role in probiotic therapy, it is unlikely to account for the wide array of beneficial effects that have been reported in other species. Alternative proposed mechanisms include antimicrobial factor production, immunoregulatory effects, anti-inflammatory effects, anticarcinogenic effects and direct effects on the intestinal mucosa. Most commercially available probiotics are certain strains of *Lactobacillus* spp, *Bifidobacterium* spp and *Enterococcus* spp. Yeasts have also been evaluated for probiotic properties, however most yeast supplements act as nutritional supplements, not probiotics. Supplementation with *Saccharomyces cerevisiae* was shown to increase intestinal yeast numbers but have no effect of bacterial counts, however supplementation of horses fed a high starch diet attenuated undesirable changes in the intestinal environment (Medina *et al.*, 2002). *Saccharomyces boulardii* has been shown to be effective for the prevention of antibiotic associated diarrhea and treatment of recurrent *Clostridium difficile* diarrhea in people (McFarland *et al.*, 1994), but its effect in horses is unclear. Yogurt is commonly used in people and animals for the treatment of enteric disease. Despite occasional anecdotal reports of success, yogurt tends to contain organisms that are poorly able to survive bile environments and are unable to colonize the intestinal tract and have much lower numbers of organisms that is likely needed to produce a beneficial effect.

Synbiotics are combinations of prebiotics and probiotics, on the theory that the prebiotics will help the probiotics survive, colonize the intestinal tract, and produce a beneficial effect.

Unfortunately, at this point marketing efforts for these products greatly exceed published research, and little information is available supporting the use of any products. There are significant quality control concerns with both human and veterinary probiotics (Weese, 2003; Weese, 2002; Hamilton-Miller and Shah, 2002) likely because nutraceuticals are unregulated in most jurisdictions. Prebiotic therapy may be a more realistic and practical approach, with a greater chance of success; however further research is required to determine the optimal prebiotic compounds and dosing regimens.

A variety of other supplements are marketed as having positive effects on the microflora. Often, a variety of substances are combined in commercial products with claims of vague effects such as "stimulant tonics to the gastrointestinal mucous membranes" and 'soothes and heals the gut". While many products claim to have research, proper research studies are almost invariably lacking and there is a heavy reliance on anecdotal reports. While the potential for some of the products having beneficial effects cannot be dismissed, there is no evidence of any beneficial effect at this time.

In general, most nutritional supplements are likely harmless even if they have no beneficial effects. The general impression of the innocuous nature of supplements should, however, not lull the equine industry into complacency because unforeseen adverse effects could be occurring. A case in point is a recent study of a probiotic (*Lactobacillus pentosus* WE7) for prevention of diarrhea in neonatal foals (Weese *et al.,* in press). Foals supplemented with this probiotic actually had a higher incidence of diarrhea, diarrhea plus other clinical abnormalities and required more veterinary examination and treatment than control foals, indicating that this specific 'pro'biotic was actually a pathogen. Adverse effects of probiotic supplementation may be more likely to occur in foals than adult horses, both because of the ability to deliver high per-kilogram doses to the small foals and because of their less developed intestinal microflora.

Intuitively, it can be suspected that *certain* prebiotics and/or probiotics could be useful for treatment or prevention of *certain* diseases, however proper research is required to identify these specific products and diseases.

Conclusion

The intestinal microflora is a vast, dynamic and poorly understood environment that is critical for the normal health and growth of horses. While the specific composition of the microflora and detailed information regarding influences on this microbial population are only superficially understood, current knowledge about effects of diseases and treatments should be used to develop appropriate management and treatment regimens to reduce (not eliminate) the risk of adverse health effects from changes in this population.

References

Baverud V., Franklin A., Gunnarsson A., *et al.*, 1998. Clostridium difficile associated with acute colitis in mares when their foals are treated with erythromycin and rifampin for Rhodococcus equi pneumonia. Equine Vet J; 30:482-488.

Dial S., Alrasadi K., Manoukian C., *et al.*, 2004. Risk of Clostridium difficile diarrhea among hospital inpatients prescribed proton pump inhibitors. CMAJ; 171:33-38.

Dwyer R.M., 2004. Environmental disinfection to control equine infectious diseases. Vet Clin North Am Equine Pract; In press.

Eckburg P.B., Bik E.M., Bernstein C.N., *et al.*, 2005. Diversity of the Human Intestinal Microbial Flora. Science 2005.

Guarner F. and Schaafsma G.J., 1998. Probiotics. Int J Food Microbiol; 39:237-238.

Gustafsson A., Baverud V., Franklin A., *et al.*, 1999. Repeated administration of trimethoprim/sulfadiazine in the horse—pharmacokinetics, plasma protein binding and influence on the intestinal microflora. J Vet Pharmacol Ther; 22:20-26.

Hamilton-Miller J.M. and Shah S., 2002. Deficiencies in microbiological quality and labelling of probiotic supplements. Int J Food Microbiol; 72:175-176.

Little D., Redding W.R., Blikslager A.T., 2001. Risk factors for reduced postoperative fecal output in horses: 37 cases (1997-1998). J Am Vet Med Assoc; 218:414-420.

McFarland L.V., Surawicz C.M., Freenberg R.N., *et al.*, 1994. A randomized placebo-controlled trial of Saccharomyces boulardii in combination with standard antibiotics for Clostridium difficile disease. J Am Med Assoc; 71:1913-1918.

Medina B., Girard I.D., Jacotot E., *et al.*, 2002. Effect of a preparation of Saccharomyces cerevisiae on microbial profiles and fermentation patterns in the large intestine of horses fed a high fiber or a high starch diet. J Anim Sci; 80:2600-2609.

Schott HC, Ewart SL, Walker RD, *et al.* 2001. An outbreak of salmonellosis among horses at a veterinary teaching hospital. J Am Vet Med Assoc; 218:1152-1159.

Van Duijkeren E., Sloet van Oldruitenborgh-Oosterbaan M.M., Houwers D.J., *et al.*, 1994. Equine salmonellosis in a Dutch veterinary teaching hospital. Vet Red; 135:248-250.

Weese J.S., 2002. Microbiologic evaluation of commercial probiotics. J Am Vet Med Assoc; 220:794-797.

Weese J.S., 2003. Evaluation of deficiencies in labeling of commercial probiotics. Can Vet J;44:982-983.

White G. and Prior S.D., 1982. Comparative effects of oral administration of trimethoprim/sulphadiazine or oxytetracycline on the faecal flora of horses. Vet Rec; 111:316-318.

Wilson D.A., MacFadden K.E., Green E.M., *et al.*, 1996. Case control and historical cohort study of diarrhea associated with administration of trimethoprim-potentiated sulphonamides to horses and ponies. J Vet Intern Med; 10:258-264.

Printed in the United States
by Baker & Taylor Publisher Services